♡
Babycalming

CAROLINE DEACON

Babycalming

Simple Solutions for a Happy Baby

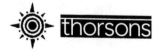

Thorsons
An Imprint of HarperCollins*Publishers*
77–85 Fulham Palace Road,
Hammersmith, London W6 8JB

The website address is www.thorsonselement.com

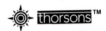

and *Thorsons* are trademarks of HarperCollins*Publishers* Ltd

First published in collaboration
with National Childbirth Trust Publishing 2004

1 3 5 7 9 10 8 6 4 2

© NCT Publishing 2004

Caroline Deacon asserts the moral right to
be identified as the author of this work

Extracts from *Dream Babies* by Christina Hardyment
(Jonathan Cape, 1983, ISBN 0-224-01910-4) are published
with kind permission of the author
© 1983 by Christina Hardyment

A catalogue record for this book
is available from the British Library

ISBN 0 00 715902 1

Printed and bound in Great Britain by
Creative Print and Design (Wales), Ebbw Vale

Contents

Acknowledgements

First and foremost I would like to thank the National Childbirth Trust. I first joined this wonderful charity 11 years ago, when I was pregnant with my first baby. The NCT gave me information, support and a new circle of friends; without it, my decisions as a parent would not have been as well informed.

I would like thank Sonia Leach, editor at NCT Publishing, for her positive and encouraging feedback and general hand-holding; Linda Griffiths, NCT Information Officer and Librarian, for tirelessly tracking down obscure research papers; Rosie Dodds, NCT Policy Research Officer, and Hilary English, NCT breastfeeding tutor, for their thoughtful contributions.

I also must thank all the parents who willingly contributed their own experiences, as well as all the breastfeeding counsellors and antenatal teachers who discussed routines, sleep and the like at study days – there are too many of you to thank individually, but you know who you are!

My biggest thanks, though, must go to my family: Mark, who has uncomplainingly put up with 11 years of NCT, babysitting through countless weekends and evenings of training, committee meetings and so on. My three children are thanked for introducing me to the endlessly fascinating world of parenting! For the colic, sleepless nights, and for enduring our endless experiments in good-enough parenting, thank you Alasdair, Chris and Josie.

Introduction – Why the Three-step Plan Works

After all the anticipation during pregnancy, when your baby finally arrives, no matter how organized you are, life will feel pretty chaotic amidst the excitement and wonder. New parents in particular are thrown straight in at the deep-end – after all, your baby doesn't come with a handy manual – and the sense of responsibility can be overwhelming.

What You Need

Like most people, you are probably used to running your life with one eye on the clock and the other on the task in hand: you have a routine and normally expect to do certain things in a certain order throughout the day. Because of this, it is natural to hope that your baby will fall into a routine that will complement yours and enable you to plan and manage your day-to-day life.

At the same time, you also hope that your baby will be happy, feed easily and sleep well. If he cries, you would like what he needs to be obvious, so that you can know how to respond. However, many babies do not appear to behave like this: they cry seemingly without reason, they sleep in fits and starts or they want to feed all the time. They don't seem to have an internal clock and they show no interest in the clock on the wall!

What Your Baby Needs

Your baby spent his first nine months being held, rocked and moved around in the womb. He was in constant contact with his mum and could hear her heartbeat, her voice, feel the warmth of her body and the sensation of being tightly held. He expected things to continue like this after birth: being in constant contact with another human being, feeling warm, snug and secure. If he thinks has been abandoned, he cries, a response that has evolved over millions of years to make sure a responsible adult picks him up and keeps him safe. If he is hungry, uncomfortable, tired or bored he will cry.

How to Help Your Baby

A psychologist called Maslow pointed out that in order for human beings to be fulfilled, reach their potential and enjoy life – 'reach self-actualization' is how he put it – they need to have their basic needs met. You can't sit and concentrate on a book or film if you are hungry, thirsty or need the toilet. Great philosophy or art will pass you by if you are homeless and worried about your safety.

Babies are like this, too – if their basic needs are not met, they cannot be happy and secure, and although there are lots of similarities between adult needs and baby needs, there are differences, too.

We all need to have enough to eat and drink, and we need to have times to rest and sleep. We all need to feel safe – for grown-ups this

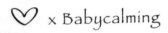 x Babycalming

might mean that the rent or mortgage is paid or that our homes are secure and we can sleep soundly at night – but for your baby, feelings about safety are a little different. Babies expect adults to fend off danger, so for your baby, safety is about human companionship. If there is a reliable grown-up nearby, then he can relax.

For your baby to feel happy and contented, you need to fulfil his three basic needs:

- **Contact**
- **Food**
- **Sleep**

Over time, the *way* you meet these needs, and the balance between them, changes. This is perhaps one of the most difficult things to grasp in parenting – the rules change all the time, and what worked today will no longer be appropriate tomorrow. Where we often go wrong is in thinking that methods stay constant.

For instance, feeding a baby whenever he is hungry, day or night, is perfectly appropriate at two weeks, but is no longer appropriate at two years. Sharing your bedroom, if not your bed, with a baby of five weeks is safe and easy; sharing your bed with a five-year-old is less easy; sharing your bed with a fifteen-year-old would certainly be odd! Responding the instant your baby cries when he is little is appropriate; responding to a toddler who is yelling for sweets is not kind in the long run.

Every healthy baby wants to communicate, will make demands and will make his presence felt. Initially, the only way he knows how to get your attention is by crying. In general, if you understand and work within his needs, he will not need to cry for prolonged periods and you and he will enjoy plenty of positive and happy times together.

This does not mean endless self-sacrifice on your behalf: normally, your needs and your baby's needs will not fundamentally conflict, because nature has designed a system that works in harmony with you both.

What This Book Can Do for You

This book is fundamentally different from the many other parenting books on the shelves. Some books cast you loose, tell you to trust your instincts and leave you to get on with it. If anything, they hope that if you respond to your baby all the time without question, he will eventually just evolve into the kind of child that you would like him to be. Most parents need more reassurance and guidance than that.

Other books – and this is a more popular approach at the moment – impose on your baby a rigid schedule from the day he is born. However, unless this particular schedule happens to suit you and your baby, you are probably both going to be unhappy with it. If it does work for you, the chances are that this is the schedule or routine you would both have arrived at anyway!

Then there is a third way, a middle way, which is to understand your baby's needs, respond to them appropriately, and to introduce the routines and boundaries your child wants – but at the right times and in a way that does not fundamentally conflict with your own needs. *Babycalming* follows this third way and shows you what is appropriate and when. It is a three-step plan based on your baby's three basic needs for contact, food and sleep, and it will also help you to devise and settle into a routine that is right for you both.

It is a combination of tried-and-tested methods from my experience as an NCT (National Childbirth Trust) breastfeeding counsellor and mother of three, and research-based evidence.

Throughout the book you will find quotations from different experts, philosophers and public figures regarding children and childcare over the last couple of centuries. They are quoted at the beginning of each chapter, then at the end you will find out when it was said. You will see that some opinions on childcare haven't changed at all, whereas others will seem completely inappropriate. They are there to remind you that opinions on childcare change all the time, and that as a parent you can only do what you think is best for your baby at the present time according to all the information and advice you have at that moment.

With this in mind, try not to worry or feel guilty if you find it over-whelming being a parent, or if you are unsure that you are doing the right thing for your baby. Instead, enjoy your baby, celebrate his presence in your life and know that if you can meet his three basic needs for contact, food, and sleep, you will be well on the way to bringing up a happy and contented baby.

♡

Your Baby from Birth to Toddlerhood

Why Do Babies Cry?

~ Times change – does the advice stay the same? ~

At no previous time has there been such a wide general interest in all that concerns childhood, as shown by the numerous books constantly issuing from the press upon these subjects and the periodicals devoted to the different phases of the child problem.

Most people can ignore all sorts of noise – the buzz of conversations, engine noises, even the radio or TV – but the instant a baby starts crying, everyone looks tense. They need it to stop.

Your baby's appearance is designed to make you want to take care of him; he has a smooth, round forehead, big eyes, a head that's large in proportion to his body – in all mammals this signals, 'I'm a baby – take care of me!' In the same way, the sound of your baby's crying is designed to make sure you attend to him – now! We all react to the sound of a baby's cry with increased heart rate, raised blood pressure and sweating – the common reactions to stress. A baby's cry is meant to be stressful, to evoke an instant response.

How Easy Is It to Tell Why Your Baby Is Crying?

Mothers quickly become tuned in to their own baby's crying, so well in fact that after only three nights in a postnatal ward, a new mother can pick out her own baby's cries *in her sleep*.[1]

However, although you will quickly learn to identify your own baby's cry, it's not like a language where such-and-such a cry means, 'I'm hungry!' while another cry means, 'I'm bored!' With most babies, what varies is only the intensity and volume of their cry, rather than its tone or content, though as your baby gets older he will be more sophisticated at letting you know what he wants.

We know this from research. In one study, researchers played two tapes to mothers: one was of a one-month-old hungry baby, the other was of a newborn baby who'd just been circumcised. When the mothers were asked whether the babies were hungry, sleepy, in pain, angry, startled or wet, only 25 per cent could correctly identify the hungry baby (40 per cent thought he was over-tired), while for the other tape, only 40 per cent could identify the pain cry correctly, with 30 per cent thinking he was startled or angry.[2] Another piece of research, from Finland, asked 80 very experienced baby nurses to listen to recordings of babies crying. Once again, even with their experience, they were correct only 50 per cent of the time.[3]

Some researchers have tried analysing babies' cries using acoustical measuring equipment. People like Barry Lester at Brown University have found that a baby's cry may be significantly different when he has certain medical conditions; for instance, a malnourished baby has a weaker cry, while babies with *cri-du-chat*, a chromosome disorder, also have a distinctive cry. However, apart from these unusual examples, it seems impossible to classify the average baby's cry as a precise language.

This does not mean it's not worth trying to understand your baby's cries! In time you probably will get to know what your baby wants, not by interpreting his cry, but by coming to know who he is, what he likes, and of course by the context: whether he has been fed recently, needs a sleep, and so on.

How the Three-step Plan Will Help

The three steps are a great way to start thinking about responding appropriately to your baby's crying. Over time, as you grow in confidence, and as you and your baby get to know each other and to learn to communicate, you will begin to learn what is wrong without any help from other people.

Am I Spoiling My Baby by Picking Him Up When He Cries?

Some people believe that picking a baby up when he cries, teaches him to cry, and this view is at the heart of many sleep programmes, as you will see later in this book. But while there is a stage at which a baby can be encouraged to fall asleep alone, a newborn who is left to cry will not feel loved and secure, just abandoned. Tiny babies are incapable of comprehending why they might have to wait, but if your baby knows his needs will be met when he cries, he will learn that he is not alone – he is loved, he can influence the world, and the world in turn is dependable (all important lessons).

Tuning In to Your Baby's Needs

Take the time to tune in to your baby and find out what he wants. You will not only have a happier baby and a good relationship, you will be encouraging his development!

Barry Lester worked with one-month-old babies, taping their cries and playing them back to their mothers, asking what was wrong.[5] He found that the babies whose mothers could interpret their cries correctly, had higher mental scores at 18 months of age and had learnt 2½ times as many words as babies whose mothers had not tuned in to their babies' cries.

'If the mother can read her baby's cues she is more likely to be providing the kind of child-rearing environment that will enrich development and facilitate cognition later on,' Lester says.[6]

Try to remember that most babies have fairly simple needs – the need to be touched, held and fed, the need to be comfortable, the need to feel safe, the need for human company and the need to sleep. They cry to let someone know there is a problem, and all they expect is that someone will deal with the problem. Your baby won't cry to annoy you, 'get at' you, or from any other complicated motive. Try to avoid projecting your own feelings onto your baby when interpreting why he's crying.

As he grows, you can encourage him to use other methods of communication by interpreting his cries verbally: 'Oh, you want a drink, do you?' If you are calm when he is agitated, he will begin to learn to calm himself and regain control. As he reaches his toddler years he is going to need to learn about 'deferred gratification', so not responding instantly to screams will do an older baby no harm, as you will see later on in this book.

Why Your Baby Might Be Crying

- **Listen to your gut feeling – what do you think your baby needs? You are probably the best person to know.**

Step One: Feeding

In the first few weeks, most mothers try feeding first. Suckling is comforting, and you cannot overfeed a breastfed baby. If you are formula feeding, you need to keep an eye on the amount your baby consumes in 24 hours, but if you're mixing feeds correctly and staying within the recommended amounts, you will not overfeed your baby.

If he is opening his mouth and turning his head ('rooting'), this is a good indication that he's hungry, so you can begin to look for these cues, and feed him even before he starts crying. We will look at why baby-led feeding is important, especially with breastfeeding, in the section on Step One, as well as looking at other ways of fulfilling your baby's need to suckle.

Step Two: Comfort

IS HE COMFORTABLE?
Check his nappy. Feel his abdomen to find whether he's too cold or hot. Is he in pain? If he is in pain, he will probably not stop crying even when you pick him up, and his crying will be intense;

high-pitched, with breath-holding in the middle – although, as we have seen earlier, it's not possible to be exact about the meaning of a particular type of cry. However, if you are at all worried, do ring your GP.

IS HE BORED?

If you've eliminated obvious physical discomfort, then your baby may be frightened, lonely or bored; i.e., in need of human company for comfort! In this case he will probably stop crying when you pick him up. You will find lots of suggestions for soothing a crying baby later on in the section on Step Two.

Paediatrician Berry Brazelton suggests that you don't rush straight in but watch instead to see whether your baby can soothe himself. He suggests six things to try in turn. First, *show your baby your face* to see if that reassures him. Then, *speak gently* to see if face and voice alone can soothe. The next method to try is *a warm hand laid gently on his tummy*; then try *both hands* to contain his arms and legs. If none of these manages to calm your baby, *pick him up*. It can be good to hold him in a position which makes him feel safe and secure (see page 79) or to wrap him up securely with access to his knuckles or fingers so that he can suck them (see page 79). Sucking is the most soothing thing for a baby.[7]

Step Three: Sleep

Is he tired? Babies are not skilled at getting themselves to sleep, and can cry through tiredness. Your baby will need lots of sleep to help him grow and learn, and there is information about ways of helping your baby to sleep in the section on Step Three, as well as how your baby's need for sleep can dovetail with yours, so you and your family get all the sleep you need.

My second baby wanted to be held a lot when he was little, and my first was just aged 20 months at the time and wanting mummy too. So I bought a second-hand baby sling from a friend and 'wore' my newborn on my front for the first couple of weeks. It kept him quiet and content and left me free to get on with everything else.

— Sonia, mother of Anna, Ricky and Jessica

~ Times Change ~ Answer – 1899 ~

Dr Holt, author of the bestselling The Care and Feeding of Children, *addressing the third annual convention of the National Congress of Mothers in Washington DC, mid-February 1899*

2

Getting Used to the World: The First Six Weeks

~ Times change – does the advice stay the same? ~

Childrearing, like cheap wine, does not travel well.

If we compare our Western culture to any other, throughout history or elsewhere in the world, we probably are the least baby-centred society ever to exist. Mothers give birth and are expected to get 'back to normal' in a matter of days. We ignore the fact that giving birth, even without complications or interventions, is the physical equivalent of running a marathon.

You Need Time

In most cultures, women are cared for by other women after birth for an average of 40 days. That's how it should be. It's a complete myth that some women give birth at the side of a field and then carry on with normal chores. 'Lying-in' after birth is the norm for most, and

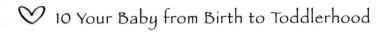

six weeks seems a sensible time to allow a mother to recover and to get to know her baby. It is a time for physical rest and for establishing a milk supply. A new mother needs a lot of support, love and care – she too, needs a lot of mothering.

Your Baby Needs Time

A newborn baby also needs time to get used to the world, to find out what is expected of her, and to get to grips with basic skills like feeding. Although there is a surprising amount that she can do for herself, she is still dependent on you and needs you to help her help herself. Take time to try the steps mentioned on page 8 before rushing in.

We are in such a rush to get on, get back to normal, get into a routine, get to the next stage ... but babies take time, especially in these first six weeks. It takes time to build up a breastmilk supply, it takes time for your baby to learn to feed. Everything is slow – but don't worry, it will speed up; in the meantime, consider this stage as a six-week baby-honeymoon or 'babymoon'!

These first six weeks are also a time for you and your baby to get to know each other, and to spend time in close contact. Other mammals bond by 'imprinting' – goats and sheep, for instance, need to be in constant contact in the first few hours and days after birth to learn who is who and to bond. We humans, too, need time spent in contact to develop that close relationship.

One writer, Tine Thevenin, has an interesting theory about how we in the West raise children. We value independence above all, she claims, which is a male value. Women, she says, are less uncomfortable with dependency, but as we live in a male-dominated society, we push our babies towards independence sooner than we should. Hence the desire to get babies to sleep alone, to be put down in cribs rather than held close.[1]

Step One: Feeding

In the first six weeks, your baby needs to feed a lot. Her tummy is only the size of a walnut, so it empties quickly. She is small and not yet practiced at feeding – it will take her some time to fill that tiny tummy. If she's breastfeeding, she has to feed often to build up a milk supply, and she relies on you to hold her in the optimum position to do this; she will not be able to alter position by herself as she can when she's older. Finally, if she is to survive, she needs to grow – she will double her weight in the first few months of life – never again will she need to grow so quickly.

At this stage, if your baby cries or seems to need something, try feeding first.

It may well feel, especially if you decide to breastfeed, that all you are doing is feeding your baby in these first six weeks. There is so much conflicting advice around feeding, but breastfeeding is really the best thing you can do for your baby

**DID YOU KNOW?
– babies need contact!**
In the 1940s, psychiatrist René Spitz compared two groups of disadvantaged babies; one group were reared in prison by their own mothers who gave them attention and affection, even though most of their time was spent in the prison nursery. Despite the deprivation of their surroundings, these babies developed normally.

The other group of babies were in an orphanage with one nurse for eight babies, and they were left in their cots, and only taken out for feeding and changing. The sides of the cots were draped with sheets to prevent the spread of infection. This meant the babies could not see out. Tragically, many of these babies did not live to two years of age, and those who did were physically stunted and severely retarded, emotionally and mentally. Few could walk or talk by age three, and they were withdrawn and apathetic.[2]

and it is worth investing your time in these early weeks to learn how to do it.

If you do feel worried that your baby is breastfeeding a lot, have a look at the guide to positioning your baby at your breast in Step One entitled Feeding Your Newborn (pages 43–4); sometimes you can improve this a little so that your baby can feed more efficiently and therefore more quickly. You could also ring a breastfeeding counsellor for help; the NCT National Breastfeeding Line is open from 8 a.m. to 10 p.m. seven days a week, tel: 0870 444 8708.

The section on Step One also explains in more detail why it is important to breastfeed your baby whenever she seems hungry. Baby-led feeding, or feeding 'on demand', is vital at this stage. Routines can and will develop – but not yet. So sit back and relax; take the time to recover from the birth, and before you know it you will be at the next stage, when you can think about schedules, routines, bottles and everything else. By six months, feeding will be only a small part of your daily life together – and by the time she's a toddler, you may find you have one of those children who is too busy with life to bother with such mundane things as meals!

Your baby will communicate her hunger by bringing her hands to her mouth and rooting – turning her head from side to side with her mouth open. It makes feeding easier if you can feed her before she cries – a crying baby is using up energy and does not always feed efficiently.

- **Try feeding first at this stage – baby-led feeding means letting her decide at this stage – which will establish your milk supply.**

Step Two: Comfort

In the early weeks your baby has an enormous amount of information to process; everything is new to her right now! Crying is her most effective communication tool at this stage, and she may fuss and cry far more at this age than at any other. As her world has changed so immensely, from being in the womb to being out in the world, perhaps this is to be expected. Your baby is often soothed by reminders of the womb: the sounds, regular movement, and by the sense of being held.

It's good to hold and soothe your baby a lot at this stage; she may be comforted by being firmly wrapped in a cot blanket (swaddled), or by rocking or being carried, and by contact with other people. She might also enjoy background noise – her Mum's voice, of course, but also 'white noise' like the washing machine, vacuum cleaner or car engine! There are lots of practical suggestions about this in the section on Step Two.

Some babies cry a huge amount, and may be labelled as having 'colic' – and we will look at this in more detail in Step Two.

- **Don't worry that your baby seems to need a lot of soothing at this stage. She will cry and fuss more now than at any other time. It will pass; in the meantime she will be comforted by contact – holding, rocking – do whatever you feel is right!**

Step Three: Sleep

She will sleep far more, too, at this early age than at any other, but her sleep will be erratic, as she has not yet grasped the difference between day and night, and may still find it difficult to soothe herself back to sleep when she wakes.

In the first six weeks her patterns will develop; she will start to learn about day and night, and you can help her by emphasizing this difference. At night, for instance, you can keep the lights low when you feed, and keep noise and interaction to a minimum. You probably won't change her nappy unless it is dirty.

As you get on top of things, you can start to introduce a bedtime routine – another part of helping her to sleep. The section on Step Three explains how sleep works, and looks at all the options for helping your baby to sleep. In the first six weeks, though, it is recommended that you share your room with your baby, and as she wakes several times in the night to feed, you may find it easiest to bedshare too.

- **Sleep comes in short bursts; room-sharing is best, bed-sharing is easier, especially for night feeds. Emphasize the difference between day and night, and start to introduce a bedtime routine as soon as you can.**

All this adds up to a lot of time spent just attending to your baby! But like every stage of parenting, it doesn't last long, and it is vital that you do spend time just concentrating on your baby in these early weeks.

My daughter Charlotte had bad colic, or at least was very windy, and we found that the best method for getting the wind up was to pat her back in three stages. First patting the bottom, then the middle, then the top of her back, as if to help the wind come up.
– Elizabeth, mother to Charlotte

~ Times Change ~ Answer – 1999 ~

From Three in a Bed *by Deborah Jackson (Bloomsbury, 1999)*

3

Learning about Routines: Six Weeks to Six Months

~ Times change – does the advice stay the same? ~

The cry of an infant should never be disregarded.
It is Nature's Voice.

For many parents, this stage is when they feel that they fall in love with their babies for the first time – and no wonder! The first smile, the first laugh, the coos and babbles – babies of this age can be adorable.

You are beginning to recover from the birth, you are feeling perhaps that you have your head above water – now is the time you can start to think about getting your life into a routine.

Sociable Babies

From birth, your baby can make facial movements, and if these are treated as smiles, then smiles they become. Babies of all cultures start smiling, even if they are blind, so this is truly something we are pre-programmed to do.

Babies can also vocalize from birth, but 'proto-conversation' or 'early conversation' also gets going around now, and continues until about six months. It may just look as if your baby is cooing and waving his hands around, but researchers have found that babies are mimicking the intonation of what will be their native tongue, and their hand movements keep time with the conversations around them. If you talk to your baby, he will listen, and when you pause, he will respond – he is making conversation!'

You may notice that your baby often stares at you now – this pro-longed eye contact is what helps mums fall in love with their babies; in fact, psychologists have called this 'obligatory looking', as babies can get 'stuck' staring at something, unable to look away!

Step One: Feeding

If you are breastfeeding, your milk supply should be well established by six weeks, and so now it is far easier to mould and adapt a feed-ing pattern to suit you and your family's needs. If you are thinking about giving your baby bottles at some stage, perhaps because you will be returning to work soon, then six weeks is a great age to intro-duce these – your baby should be able to adapt to the new sucking technique without it interfering with his ability to breastfeed.

By now you may see some sort of pattern to your baby's feeding, and you can perhaps start to negotiate a routine that would suit you better. Perhaps you would like him to feed a little longer in the afternoon and early evening so he may go longer between feeds at night. If he is a very 'suckly' baby, let him suck his fingers or thumbs, or you might want to introduce a dummy – have a look at the chapter called Your Baby's Need to Suckle (page 59) for more on this.

He will still rely just on breastmilk or formula for nutrition at this stage; the latest research suggests that there is no benefit, and perhaps some disadvantage, in introducing solids before six months.[2] If your baby suddenly seems very hungry, it may well be that he is going through an 'appetite spurt' – this is where your baby feeds a lot for a short space of time to increase the milk supply – it's a bit like changing gear in a car!

Sometimes a period of intense feeding happens just before your baby falls ill, and research now suggests that babies can alert their mothers' immune system to any germs they have picked up, by leaving these on the breast skin. The breastmilk will then convey the appropriate antibodies in the next feed. Amazing!

- **Feeding at this stage should begin to fall into a pattern; it will be easier to space feeds out and predict things now. There will still be times when your baby feeds a lot – usually due to illness or a growth spurt. Solids are not recommended at this stage, but if you'd like your baby to learn how to feed from a bottle, now is a good time to introduce one.**
- **By now you will probably be learning to read your baby's cues and can tell when he is hungry. If he cries, therefore, you might try comforting him in other ways than feeding.**

Step Two: Comfort

At this stage, your baby will still fuss and cry a lot: time spent crying reaches a peak at around six weeks and declines by three or four months. Rocking, carrying and the techniques we looked at for the first six weeks will still work now. In fact at around six months, your baby's vestibular system (which detects movement and gravity, so it's how we keep our sense of balance) is at its most sensitive, and it is good to stimulate it through movement. That's why many babies love those baby-bouncers you can hang in the doorway. Older children, too, love swings and roundabouts for the same reason, because they stimulate their sense of balance and co-ordination.

Although your baby at six weeks is developing social skills and interacting with you, he is still very dependent, easily tired or over-stimulated, and fussing or colicky behaviour will be common. That's why routines can help; if your baby begins to perceive a predictable pattern to his day, it means he has less to cope with, less to take in. If your baby fusses a lot, have another look at Step Two (pages 65–112) for detailed suggestions on soothing him, and also pages 83–112 for information about colic.

Your baby's favourite sound at this age is 'motherese',[3] which is that special, high-pitched, nonsense, singsong language women use when they talk to babies. You might feel daft doing this, but you will probably find it comes naturally, and babies love it. It helps them, in turn, learn to speak far more easily!

MUM, I'M BORED! ENTERTAINING YOUR BABY
Even tiny babies are intelligent, capable human beings, and they are skilled at forming relationships. Babies hate being bored, just like the rest of us, and once they have got over the birth and initial settling into the world, they don't want to be tucked up in a cot all day: they want to get out and mix with people.

It doesn't mean you have to spend hours waving rattles in his face, but tiptoeing around a quiet house to let him sleep does nothing for the baby who wants noise and action. Let him be where he can see you and enjoy your company. Prop him somewhere safe where he can watch you do things; chat to him and tell him what you're up to. You can hang a mobile where he can look at it. Watching you, though, is often what he loves best!

Of course your baby will love it when you do find time to play with him. Repetitive games, especially where he has to respond and interact, like peek-a-boo or round and round the garden, will not only be his favourites, they also help him lay down the building blocks for the acquisition of language.

- **You are still going to be spending a lot of time at this stage, soothing your baby, in similar ways to the first six weeks. As the first few months pass, you will find this gets easier. Predictable routines may help both of you cope with the day.**

Step Three: Sleep

It is still safer to share a room with your baby at this stage, and it's also safe to share a bed as long as you're careful (see page 174). You will be hoping that he might begin sleeping through the night.

The first step towards this is to help your baby fall asleep on his own in the evenings, so if you haven't yet started a bedtime routine, you might like to look at how to do this in Step Three (pages 137–43).

The next step is to help your baby fall back to sleep on his own during the night – and there are lots of ideas about this in the section on Step Three, too. This is also the time to establish a pattern of daytime naps, so that your baby has definite times for being asleep and being awake, rather than drifting between states as he did in his first six weeks.

- **At this stage, sleeping will still mean room-sharing and perhaps bed-sharing. However, your baby should be developing the skills to help him sleep for longer periods; hopefully you will be settling him to sleep on his own, and helping him develop self-soothing techniques so that he can get back to sleep again when he wakes.**

DID YOU KNOW?
– back to sleep, but put him on his front, too!

Until your baby is rolling over by himself, you still need to put him on his back to sleep. However, recent research suggests that because babies are spending longer on their backs now due to the Back to Sleep Campaign, they are having less tummy-lying so they are slower to roll over, sit, crawl, or pull to stand than babies who used to sleep on their stomachs, although it's still within normal range. It's worth thinking about giving your baby a variety of positions during waking hours.[4]

Our first baby, Summer, had severe colic for six months; we were starting to think it would never end, and then eventually it subsided. We even took her to the doctor after four months of it, to have her checked for something more serious as we couldn't believe that colic could cause this much pain to a baby.

It started about 4 p.m. each day and went on until midnight or more. The sound of her screams and crying were so unbearable, it sounded at times as if we were beating the life out of her or something terrible – it was just pure torture. As parents, we felt so helpless – it was horrendous. We went through truckloads of Infacol, gripe water, colic drops, etc. but nothing helped. We tried endless amounts of baby massage, which sometimes soothed her a bit, as did a hot bath, and both of these things made us feel at least like we were doing something constructive to ease her pain.

– *Stephanie, mother to Summer and Eva*

~ Times Change ~ Answer – 1825 ~

From Domestic Duties *by Mrs Parkes, cited in Christina Hardyment,*
Dream Babies: Child-care From Locke to Spock (*Jonathan Cape, 1983*)

4

Getting Sociable: Six Months to Two Years

~ Times change – does the advice stay the same? ~
It is very common practice to leave a baby crying for hours on end in his pram outside the house, with nothing to do but a brick wall to see, when all he wants is something to watch.

For many parents, this stage of babyhood feels like the easiest. Your baby can sit up, but can't move about too much yet. She can play with toys to a limited extent, and at around nine months[1] she develops the ability to grasp objects between her fingers and thumb, so she gets pretty good at playing with her toys. Many parents don't really notice this ability emerging, but the use of the opposing thumb is one of the most important evolutionary developments that sets us apart from other apes.

Now she really feels strong affection for you and for all her immediate family, but this means she hates separation, and it also means she is scared of strangers. One theory about 'fear of strangers' is that it serves the same sort of function as imprinting in ducklings. Baby ducks are impelled to follow the first animal they catch sight of straight after hatching (usually, of course, this is their Mum), but human babies can't walk at birth, so they have developed another way of staying safe. Their method is to make a loud noise when they're little so that an adult will pick them up and keep them safe. Their cooing and smiling then seduces that adult into wanting to stay near.

At around eight months, however, babies develop the ability to move and might start to crawl away; that's when the fear of strangers emerges, thereby keeping a baby safe by ensuring that she will not want to lose sight of her parent.

> *Of course the problem for you is that this deep attachment/fear of strangers is probably happening at the same time as you are returning to work! It is worth pre-empting this by ensuring that your baby gets used to your child carer long before you return; perhaps, if possible, before the fear of strangers really takes hold.*

Your baby at this stage is amenable, sociable and usually content if her three needs are met. These needs are perhaps easiest to meet at this stage. Her higher brain is maturing, so she is beginning to learn self-control, as well as making more sense of what is going on around her. She might cry briefly to attract your attention, but then she will stop and wait for your response.

Step One: Feeding

Feeds are becoming far more regular, and you will be introducing solids, so her intake of food is beginning to tune in with your own. You will now start to work towards three main meals of milk plus some solids, as well as between-meal milk feeds, and a late-night feed. She might need the occasional feed for comfort in an emergency, but comfort, on the whole, will mostly come from a cuddle with a favourite person.

This is one of the most adventurous times of your baby's gastronomic life, so make the most of it! By the time she is mobile, she may become fussy about what she eats, so it is worth introducing a variety of tastes into her diet at this stage.

Step Two: Comfort

ATTACHMENT OBJECTS OR 'CUDDLIES'

Many new parents dislike the idea of a bit of cloth or a soft toy as an attachment object, but children may choose one themselves if you don't find one for them. My first baby never chose a cuddly, my second, fortunately, became attached to a particular

pillowcase cover (one of three), but my third baby selected a toy squirrel – a gift from Finland. We went through hell trying to find a replacement when 'Bobby' went missing!

If you are keen to chose an appropriate attachment object for your baby, make sure it has no buttons for eyes or nose, that there are no removable pieces of fabric, and that it is small and easy to hold and manipulate.

The soothing strategies you used in the first six months are less effective now, but also less necessary. Now she may well be content to know you are near; she may need less holding and carrying for comforting; carrying becomes instead a more efficient way of getting around the world – it gives her a better view!

It's fine to hold and carry your baby if you want to and can manage it; research seems to suggest that the more you meet your baby's needs at this age, the more independent she will be when she's older.[3] Often a quick cuddle, though, will soothe her. Her reasons for crying might be more obvious at this age, although of course this is the time when teeth erupt, which most babies seem to find pretty uncomfortable, and many want to increase milk feeds when teeth are bothering them.

DID YOU KNOW?
– carrying your child may make her brainier!
Don't worry if you seem to spend time carrying and jiggling your baby – you are helping her vestibular system develop, which is important, not only for balance, walking and general movement, but for general intelligence. Children with learning difficulties often have vestibular deficits – their sense of balance and co-ordination is often under-par.[4]
In one study, researchers compared babies who had regular sessions being swung in different positions at regular intervals to stimulate their balance system, with babies who did not receive this extra treatment, and found that the babies with the extra stimulation were more advanced in their motor skills like sitting, crawling, standing and walking.[5]

Step Three: Sleep

Your baby should by now have a settled sleep pattern, day and night. Her sleep cycle is now similar to yours, she is capable of sleeping deeply, and most sleep positions are safe now, although she should still not have a duvet or pillows. Now is a good time, therefore, to move her into her own room if that is what you want to do. She should have a good bedtime and night-time routine, as well as a good routine of daytime naps.

- **The three steps are really only a way of thinking about your day at this stage, in that she should have regular daytime naps, a good bedtime routine, and should be able to sleep through the night without disturbing you. You can move her into her own room if you want. Comforting at this stage should be relatively easy, and feeding will start to tune in to your own meal times, although of course there will still be lots of between-meal milk feeds.**

Samuel seemed to be a very 'suckly' baby, so the first few weeks were extremely taxing and challenging, trying to work out if the cry was for feed or comfort. After about four weeks I decided to try a dummy, despite being so opposed to them pre-baby. The result was amazing and I was able to eat a meal without constantly having to pick him up. Fantastic! I only used it when I felt sure the cry was for comfort, and I didn't use it at night to begin with, but after a couple of months I decided to use it after his bath and feed just to get him off to sleep. It worked, as he would spit it out once off to sleep.

At six months I decided to dispose of the dummy, as I was paranoid that he would come to rely on it and had visions of him walking around at the age of four with it stuck in his mouth – my worst nightmare. I wanted to lose it while he wasn't too aware of it. Not a problem. A few crying instances, which at the worst lasted 15 minutes, and after that he had no trouble falling off to sleep.

– Andrea, mother to Samuel

~ Times Change ~ Answer – 1954 ~

From Babies and Young Children *by Ronald and Cynthia Illingworth, as quoted in Christina Hardyment,* Dream Babies: Child-care from Locke to Spock *(Jonathan Cape, 1983)*

5

The Need for Boundaries: You and Your Toddler

~ **Times change – does the advice stay the same?** ~

Western civilizations are unique in the amount of physical separateness which they impose on infants, inventing innumerable gadgets – prams, cots, babychairs and bouncers … In other times and other parts of the world it would be dangerous to put them down for more than a moment.

It comes as a bit of a shock when that deliciously amenable baby, who smiles whenever he sees you, turns into a raging, bad-tempered toddler, who throws tantrums, refuses to go to bed and turns his nose up at everything you offer him to eat, or refuses to sit still long enough to get any food inside him! Unfortunately, none of the experts agrees about how to handle a toddler; as with all childcare, you need to pick and choose your own solution, depending on the situation and your child.

Times Change – Opinions Change

As you might have noticed from the quotes at the beginning of each chapter, opinions about raising children change from generation to generation. At the turn of the last century, it was very clear how children should behave – they were to be seen and not heard; and it was equally clear what to do if they misbehaved: 'spare the rod and spoil the child.' Victorian children, it would seem, needed taming by force and fear. By the time our parents were born, post-war but pre-flower power, physical violence had eased, but children were still treated roughly – spanking and leaving them to cry were seen as 'character building'.

By the 1970s and 1980s, ideas had changed completely, and children were brought up in a culture where feelings were beginning to be seen as paramount. Parents were to be child-centred, and smacking was no longer seen as acceptable. Tantrums, food fads, bedtime terrors – all behaviour was examined sympathetically, from the child's point of view.

The child's point of view is still important, but most people would also now agree that toddlers need firm boundaries.

This, I think, is one of the hardest things about parenting: the rules change all the time! It is hard to adjust to a life of limit-setting after a year of responding to your baby's needs, especially if, for instance, you picked him up whenever he cried, or fed him whenever he seemed hungry. But current thinking is that children flourish under a well-regulated, consistent regime, which is firm but fair.[1] After all, adults have to follow rules; if laws changed every day, you would feel confused, too.

However, many parents still worry about disciplining their children because they don't want to suppress natural exuberance, or resort to smacking – it can be hard to know where the middle line is. What you need to think about is where your boundaries or limits are, and whether these are reasonable and enforceable. Then you can agree them with your partner, and try to stick to them. If you can agree together what is acceptable and what isn't, then in the long run your child will feel secure within your firm boundaries and will not need to 'test the limits' continually with challenging behaviour.

Step One: Feeding

By the time your child is toddling, he will be eating, like you – three meals a day – but as his stomach is still small and as his energy needs are great, you will also be providing healthy snacks between meals. Toddlers still need milk drinks – and it is perfectly normal, if not common in our society, to breastfeed a toddler if you and he are happy to continue.

Food fads may start to emerge at this age; again, this is normal. Consider what nature intended: babies who can't move will have food chosen for them by a dependable adult, and they are therefore quite happy to eat whatever they are given. However, once they can move independently, they are at risk of eating harmful foods they pick up themselves, and so it makes sense for them to narrow their tastes, restricting their palates to what is already familiar; and this is what seems to happen.

That is why it is worth trying to get your child used to a varied diet *before* he is toddling.

If your toddler is a faddy eater, try not to let it bother you too much. As he is at the stage where he likes to push at boundaries, if food appears to be a big deal, he may well become choosy just for the sense of control. A few simple rules are worth thinking about, like no

pudding until he has finished his vegetables, or no coming back to the table once he has got down – whatever suits you and your family. But don't force him to eat more than he seems to want – even if he has only eaten a tiny amount. A good principle in life is not to eat past the point of repletion – after all, there are far more tubby people out there than skinny ones!

Step Two: Comfort

Many toddlers are too busy for cuddles; a toddler who starts to cling to his parents is usually one who is tired or hungry. If he comes to you for comfort, he certainly needs it; so let your child be a 'cry baby'. All children, girls and boys, need to be allowed the natural healing process of tears. It's a pity that they soon learn not to cry when they pick up what is 'acceptable' behaviour at school.

However, crying for toddlers usually means tantrums. Tantrums are normal behaviour at this developmental stage, and children have different reasons for losing their cool. Perhaps, therefore, we have to respond as we see fit on each occasion. Try not to let your toddler get overtired, and look out for signs of trouble brewing in advance, so you can head tantrums off.[2]

DISTRACTION RATHER THAN CONFRONTATION

If a confrontation develops, before you say no, think about how seriously you mean it. Try not to respond off the cuff. If the answer has to be no, you can still use distraction and negotiation, even while the bottom line is definitely no.

Say your toddler is demanding a chocolate biscuit just before dinner. You could distract him by pointing out that his favourite TV show is just starting, and by the time it's finished, dinner should be ready. If he can hang on till then, he can have the chocolate biscuit for pudding. Toddlers need to learn delayed gratification, but they need help, too!

TANTRUM FACTS
- **Children have tantrums only when they are with close family.[5]**
- **About half of all two-year-olds have tantrums almost daily.[6]**

Step Three: Sleep

Hopefully, by this stage your baby is mostly sleeping through the night, and having a couple of good naps during the day. Have a look at Step 3 (pages 113–182) if there are issues for your family now. However, often when children start to move, they also start to battle about bedtimes, and the chapter called Can You Train Your Baby to Sleep Through the Night? (page 128) looks at this in more detail.

DID YOU KNOW?
– you can't spoil a baby!

Lots of people might suggest that picking your baby up when he cries will spoil him. However, in a study which has been quoted frequently, researchers studied 26 mother-and-baby pairs over a long period of time, and found that babies whose mothers responded quickly and consistently to their cries when they were babies, cried less when they were one year of age, than those whose mothers had ignored their cries.[3]

These findings are so interesting and seem so significant, that another researcher recently followed this up with a larger experiment. She looked at over 100 babies over four years, and this time worked with families where mothers might not normally be responsive to their babies' cries. In some, experimenters taught the mothers to respond to the babies' cries – the rest were 'control' families. The researchers found that in families where mothers were more responsive, the babies actually cried less.[4]

Supermarkets have become a no-go zone. I hate it. Now I either leave them at home, or get Daddy to do the shopping. I simply can't get round a supermarket with all of them in tow. As far as tantrums in general go, my initial reaction used to be to lose my temper, though I knew this was unhelpful. Now I tend to go quiet and walk away. I reckon, 'This is going to resolve itself, and doesn't need me to add fuel to the fire.'

— *Katherine, mother of Hugh, Thomas, Megan and Gareth*

~ Times Change ~ Answer – 1981 ~

From Babyhood *by Penelope Leach (2nd edn; Penguin)*

Putting the

Three-step

Plan to Work

♡

Feeding

6

Feeding Your Newborn

~ Times change – does the advice stay the same? ~
*The lungs do not expand to their full extent unless they are
exercised every day. The infant has to cry – if nature is regularly
thwarted by some well-meaning person who picks up the baby,
there is a risk of the lungs remaining almost unexpanded.*

During the first few weeks you will spend a lot of time feeding your
baby. Treat it as an apprenticeship and, before you know it, you and
your baby will be old hands at it. In this chapter we'll look at the
mechanics of feeding; the following chapter will look at how much
and how often to feed your baby in the early weeks.

Bottle-feeding – How to Do It

There is a huge choice in formula-feeds – it can be difficult to decide
what to buy. You will need at least six bottles and teats, some method
of sterilizing, plus of course the formula.

It is probably best to be guided by your midwife and health visitor about which formula to start your baby on. She should also run through with you, at least once, how to prepare a bottle – but you must make sure that you read the instructions on the tin carefully, as it is important that the ratio of water to powder is correct. Don't ever be tempted to make the milk thinner or thicker than instructed.

Bottle Feeding – A Step-by-Step Guide

1 Sterilize everything you are going to use – bottles, teats, measures, knife.
2 Boil more water than you need, and allow it to cool.
3 Fill each bottle to the correct level, using the cooled boiled water.
4 Using the spoon provided in the tin of formula, take a scoop of formula and level it with the knife. Don't pat it down.
5 Add the powder to the bottle, put the top on and shake thoroughly.
6 Place in fridge until you want to use it.
7 When you want to feed the bottle to your baby, heat it by placing it in a jug of hot water. Test the temperature by shaking a few drops onto the skin in the crook of your arm, or the inside of your forearm.
8 Sit comfortably and hold your baby across your lap, sitting her a little upright if you can.
9 Keep the bottle at an angle, so the teat is full, to avoid air bubbles.

Breastfeeding – How to Do It

Have you ever wondered why it's called 'breastfeeding' not 'nipple feeding'? Because your baby feeds from a mouth full of breast – she doesn't suck on your nipples. In fact, she needs a large enough mouthful so that your nipple comes into contact with her soft palate, which is at the back of the roof of her mouth.

When your baby's soft palate is stimulated, she instinctively starts to move her jaws so that she can breastfeed. If your nipple is not far enough in, it makes contact instead with your baby's hard palate; peek in her mouth and you will see ridges. Your nipple would soon get sore pressed into that part of your baby's mouth.

As with bottle-feeding, someone should be there to help you the first few times you try to feed your baby, but these are the general principles:

Before you begin, get comfy. You could be sitting in the same position for quite a while! It's easier in the beginning to sit upright, so choose a chair which will support you sitting upright rather than slouching back, as this tends to pull your breast out of your baby's mouth. You might need cushions or pillows to help you get upright.

Your feet should reach the floor so that your knees are level or even slightly raised, to give your baby a nice cosy lap. A small stool or some telephone directories under your feet may help.

If your breasts are high then you might find a pillow or even two useful to rest your arms on when bringing your baby level with your breasts. It's easier to get your baby latched on first, and then tuck the pillows under your arms, otherwise the pillows can get between the two of you when you are trying to get started.

The most common position for holding a baby is across your tummy, but you could hold her 'underarm', especially if she's small, or if you've had a caesarean section and you need to protect your tummy. You will need to have several cushions between you and the chair back if feeding underarm, so your baby can stretch out without pushing herself off your breast. If she's across your tummy, support her head on your forearm (not the crook of your arm).

Top Tips for Correct Positioning at the Breast

- *Support your baby's spine in line.* Hold her so her back and shoulders are straight. Avoid holding the back of her head, which would push her chin towards her chest, making it difficult for her to open her mouth wide. Also, most babies don't like having their heads held.
- *Hold your baby so you are both tummy to tummy.* She will not be able to feed well if she has to turn her head sideways.
- *Align your baby's head so she's nose to nipple.* Don't hold her mouth to your nipple, as would seem logical, because once she's on your breast, her chin would be pushed

DID YOU KNOW?
Who is in control of feeding and appetite? It depends whether your baby is breastfed or bottle-fed. With a bottle, you fill it up and you can watch it empty. If you're breastfeeding, you can't tell how much your baby has had to eat and so you have to rely on your baby's signals to work out when she has had enough.

The significance of this is that breastfeeding babies are more in control of their feeds, and their mothers need to tune in to their needs. Researchers have found that bottle-feeding mothers are more likely to override cues, ignoring signals which tell them that their baby has had enough to eat.[1]

Babies, whether breastfed or bottle-fed, do not suck continuously, but have frequent breaks to be winded or have nappies changed and so on. One researcher filmed mothers feeding their babies to see who initiated these breaks, and found that it's the mother who controls the breaks for bottle-fed babies, while pauses in breastfeeding are controlled by the baby.[2]

towards her chest and her throat would close, making swallowing difficult and slow. Your nipple needs to be in contact with the roof of her mouth for her to feed properly, and needs to be far enough back to avoid contact with her hard palate – that bony ridge at the front of her mouth, which would rub against and hurt your nipple.

- *Wait for the gape.* Wait until her mouth is really wide open – imagine she's about to bite on an apple – and then draw her swiftly onto your breast.
- *Chin in.* Her chin will contact your breast first, digging well in, and leaving her nose clear.

My second child, Eva, is 12 weeks old and all afternoon she wants to be rocked and carried; it's the only way to calm her down. I wish I had some magic advice to offer, but I don't. All I can say is, if you have family or friends close by who are willing to come and pace the floor rocking your baby, ask them. I leave her with my mum while I go food shopping. It gets me out of the house for an hour and gives me a break at least from the crying.

- *Stephanie, mother of Summer and Eva*

~ Times Change ~ Answer – 1922 ~

From Charis Ursula Frankenburg, Common Sense in the Nursery *(reprinted 1934, 1954), cited in Christina Hardyment,* Dream Babies: Child-care From Locke to Spock *(Jonathan Cape, 1983)*

7

How Much
and How Often?

~ Times change – does the advice stay the same? ~

*Breastmilk is poured forth from an exuberant overflowing Urn, by a
bountiful hand, that never provides sparingly. Thus Nature, if she
be not interrupted, will do the whole business perfectly well.*

Long ago, babies were carried around all the time and fed whenever they seemed hungry. This century, lots of feeding regimes have
come and gone, so now many mothers feel completely confused
about what babies want or need. Add to this conflicting advice from
mothers, grandmothers, aunts and possibly even midwives, GPs
and health visitors, and it's no wonder women feel a bit lost as to
what's best.

For instance, a generation ago mothers were told to feed babies for
20 minutes only, every four hours. Although we now know that this
led to a downturn in breastfeeding rates, many books still try to suggest new time limits, new regimes for breastfeeding.

The advice is always well meant; the 'expert' hopes to make life for a new mother easier by imposing routines on baby from day one. For some mothers and babies, this will work, but for others feeding won't work like this, the baby will be unhappy, he may not gain weight, and breastfeeding will eventually fail.

One of the reasons that bottle-feeding can seem attractive is that mothers know exactly what they are giving their babies and when. Breastfeeding can seem a bit of an inexact science in comparison. With bottle-feeding, it is perfectly possible to schedule feeds from birth.

Bottle-feeding

If you have decided to bottle-feed your baby, you will find the question of how much and how often relatively easy, as it is all printed on the side of the tin. You and your baby may be happy to feed according to a schedule – so many ounces at certain times of the day; however, some babies will not like feeding like this, and so it's OK to bottle-feed on demand – just like breastfeeding. You need to have some way of keeping a record of exactly how much your baby takes at each feed, so that you can ensure he is getting all he needs in any 24 hour period.

Rather than continue to feed your baby when he has had the amount recommended, you will probably have to comfort him in other ways. Bottle-fed babies are usually quite happy to take a dummy, as the sucking technique is the same. Have a look at the chapter called Your Baby's Need to Suckle for more about the pros and cons of using dummies. The section on Step Two (pages 65–111) also has lots of suggestions about calming and comforting your baby without feeding him.

Breastfeeding

Breastfeeding is really very different from bottle-feeding in the first few weeks, and it is best to put all ideas about schedules out of your head for that time. Be assured that your baby will develop a feeding pattern and that it will become easier to establish a routine; the problems occur when you try to establish a clock-governed routine in the first six weeks.

WHY DOES EARLY SCHEDULE-FEEDING FAIL FOR SOME BABIES?

Trying to Go Too Long Between Feeds
The first suggestion you might hear is to try to 'space feeds out' – the idea being that you can store up milk and also get your baby to be really hungry so he will take more at a feed.

Unfortunately, breasts are not like taps; milk is not just produced when the baby feeds. Breastmilk is being made all the time, and stored between feeds in the breast. How much is made depends on how full the breast is. If the baby does not feed very often, then the breasts will fill and milk production will decrease.

Recent research has also found that women vary enormously in their storage capacity; with one woman able to store 300 per cent more than another woman, for instance, and this capacity has nothing to do with breast size. All women are capable of producing the same amount of milk over 24 hours, but women who have larger storage capacities can go longer between feeds and still give their babies enough to eat, while others will need to feed more often to deliver the same amount of milk to their babies.[1]

Women with larger storage capacities might well be able to schedule feed – but, ironically, the chances are that their babies will go for

longer between feeds anyway! Problems happen for those with small-er capacity, where stretching feeds will ultimately result in less milk being produced in 24 hours.

During pregnancy, lots of milk-making cells are created inside the breast – more than your baby is likely to need. In the early weeks after birth, some of those milk-making cells will be switched on, the rest switched off according to how frequently your baby feeds. While this is happening, your milk supply is kept high by the hormone *pro-lactin*, but after a few weeks, once your body reckons it knows how many milk-producing cells it will need for your baby, the prolactin levels decline.

This is why some mothers and babies seem to manage to breastfeed by schedule initially, but have problems later. Their bodies did pro-duce enough milk when their prolactin levels were high, but limiting the frequency of feeds led to many of the milk-producing cells being 'switched off' so that eventually the milk levels declined below what their baby needed.[2]

The final problem with trying to space feeds out is that a newborn who is crying with hunger, even for a few minutes, can find latching on and suckling more difficult than a baby who is put straight to the breast when he seems hungry. The idea that he will take more at each feed because he's hungry is erroneous; instead, if he uses up energy crying and being stressed at waiting to feed, he will take less milk at a feed and so, in time, the milk supply will decrease.[3]

Trying to Restrict Time at the Breast
The other suggestion you might hear is to try to limit your baby's time during a feed. However, there are problems with this too ...

A breastfeed starts with *fore milk* (the milk which comes in *before*), which is dilute and thirst-quenching, and gradually thickens into *hind milk* (the milk which follows *behind*), which is packed with calories. So, when your baby latches on, first he has a refreshing drink, then he gets down to a satisfying meal of hind milk, which helps him grow at an enormous rate.

Therefore, if you limit your baby's time at the breast, or swap sides too soon, he won't get so much of the hind milk he needs to grow, so he will be hungry again very quickly.

FEED YOUR BABY ON DEMAND – IT'S NATURAL!

Only your baby knows how hungry he is, and how much breastmilk he needs to grow properly. If you think about it, this is how you feed, too. Your body tells you when you are hungry, when you are thirsty, and when you are full up. You can go to the fridge and help yourself; your baby has to signal to you to put him to your breast, and he will come off when he's had enough.

It can help with worries about how long your baby takes over his feeds if again you think about the adult he will grow up to be. Sometimes we have a quick snack, or just a little drink; sometimes we are really hungry and will enjoy a big scoff. Occasionally we go out to a restaurant and sit for a few hours, enjoying a meal with friends. How would it be if the waiter rushed up and said, 'Right, you have had 20 minutes, you must have finished by now'?

COMFORT FEEDING

Some mothers worry that their baby is 'just comfort feeding'. They wonder how they can tell when he's breastfeeding because he's hungry, and when he's feeding for other reasons. Again, think about yourself. How many of those chocolate biscuits or cups of coffee do you have because you are hungry or thirsty, and how many do you have for 'comfort'? Do you only eat and drink at meal times and because you really need to, or do you sometimes have meals or snacks to be sociable, or to relieve boredom?

 50 Step One: Feeding

For a baby, breastfeeding is not just about nutrition, it is also about warmth and closeness and learning to be a social human being. Researchers notice that breastfeeding babies interact with their mums, pausing while she talks to break off feeds and listen, then replying by sucking. The belief is that feeding forms an important part of learning to make conversation – the start of social interaction.

Try not to feel pressured into feeding your baby according to someone else's idea of the right pattern. If you feel happy with the way breast-feeding is going, and if your baby is healthy and growing, then you are doing everything right. Remember, you can't spoil a baby, or overfeed him. If you feel unhappy with feeding – perhaps you don't like feed-ing him as much as it seems he wants to – then talk it through with a breastfeeding counsellor. She won't tell you what you 'must' do or put added pressure on you, but will help you explore your options so you can feel right in doing what you want to do. Sometimes she can suggest altering the way you hold your baby, so that feeding can be more efficient – see the previous chapter for more about positioning.

SUCCESSFUL BREASTFEEDING IN THE EARLY WEEKS
- **Feed as often as your baby asks.**
- **Feed for as long as your baby wants.**

Once your milk supply is established at the levels your baby needs, you will begin to see a pattern to his feeds, and then it becomes easier to negotiate a routine.

Having a baby is a real shock to the system. I certainly reacted by reading lots and lots of childcare books. (If all else fails, please read the instructions!) But to many, putting a tiny baby onto a strict routine (rather than following your instinct in fulfilling the child's need) is a robotic style of parenting that deprives you of some of the real pleasures of motherhood. My six months' maternity leave was the first time in my life I did NOT have to follow a routine, and it was very enjoyable. My son did learn the difference between night and day (automatic when they share your bed and see you asleep at night), and he did develop a routine.

– *Mette, mother of Samuel.*

~ Times Change ~ Answer – 1748 ~

From Essay on Nursing *by William Cadogan, as quoted in Christina Hardyment,* Dream Babies: Child-care From Locke to Spock
(*Jonathan Cape, 1983*)

8

Night-feeding

~ Times change – does the advice stay the same? ~

*Breastfeeding may have been natural, but we don't live in that time
now and we must adapt. Let no mother condemn herself to be a
common or ordinary 'cow' – women have not the stamina they once
possessed, and I myself know of no greater misery than nursing a
child, the physical collapse caused by which is often at the bottom
of the drinking habits of which we hear so much.*

As we saw in the previous chapter, breastfeeding your baby whenever she seems hungry is important in those early weeks. If you are
bottle-feeding, you will probably also find it more satisfying to feed
on demand.

Why Does Your Baby Need to Feed at Night?

BENEFITS FOR YOUR BABY
- Your baby needs milk at night because she simply can't store enough food during the day to keep her going.
- Feeding at night is comforting, helping her get back to sleep.

BENEFITS FOR MUM
- Breastfeeding at night in the early weeks helps your milk supply get established. The more you feed, the higher your prolactin levels, and therefore the more milk you will make.
- When you breastfeed at night, your body releases dopamine, which is soporific – it helps you get back to sleep; a big advantage over bottle-feeding.[1]

Bottle-feeding at night

If you are formula-feeding, you will still need to feed your baby at night. The easiest way to do this is to sterilize a thermos flask as well as your baby's feeding bottle and teat. Put the required measure of formula in the feeding bottle without adding the water, and seal it. Then boil some water, let it cool to just above body temperature, and put it in the thermos flask. You can then add the warm water to the feeding bottle when your baby wakes at night, thus quickly and easily preparing formula at the right temperature, without having to spend ages heating bottles.

If you need more than one bottle – which you certainly will in these early weeks – put the right amount of formula powder in each bottle and have enough heated water in the thermos for all of them.

*What you must **not** do is keep prepared formula warm, or re-use heated formula when he wakes again.*

Breast or Formula – Which Is Easier at Night?

Most researchers agree that bottle-fed babies stop feeding in the early hours of the morning at an earlier age than breastfeeding babies; usually dropping those feeds at around 10 weeks compared to 16 weeks.[2] As time goes on, breastfed babies carry on waking more frequently than bottle-fed babies. This makes bottle-feeding at night seem like an attractive option, but it is worth thinking first about the reasons why there are these differences:

- **Formula milk takes longer to digest. Because breastmilk is ideally designed for your baby, it is digested more easily than formula.**
- **Breastfed babies wake more often because they have come to expect their mothers to be more responsive. Breastfed babies are in control of how much and how often they feed, and breastfeeding mothers will respond to their babies' feeding cues rather than deciding when it is time to feed according to the directions on the tin of formula. The upside of this is that breastfed babies are less likely to have weight problems later on.[3]**
- **It may also mean your baby will be more intelligent! We already know that breastfed babies have higher average IQs than formula-fed babies; this may be partly due to the long-chain fatty acids in breastmilk, but it could also be due to breastfeeding on demand allowing your baby to have 'mastery' over her environment – a key element in cognitive development.[4]**
- **The final reason may simply be that breastfeeding is easier to do than bottle-feeding, so breastfeeding mothers feel less inclined to try to get their babies to sleep through the night, particularly if they are co-sleeping.**

Of course, this is comparing a flexibly-fed breastfed baby with a baby fed on formula according to a fixed schedule. If you are formula-feeding on demand and responding to your baby's needs rather than to the clock, it may also be that your baby follows a similar night-feeding pattern to a breastfed baby; we don't know, as the research has not been done.

An Easier Time of It

Co-sleeping breastfeeding mothers have an easier time of it than non-co-sleeping, bottle-feeding mothers. Breastfeeding at night, particularly in the early weeks, can be easier if your baby is in bed with you; the chapter called Who Sleeps Where? goes into this in more detail. Once you both have got the hang of feeding lying down, you will find that you barely wake up when she feeds, and that it's more restful than getting out of bed.

DID YOU KNOW?
– Sleeping and breastfeeding work together

Helen Ball is doing research into co-sleeping in northeast England, and has found that[5] breastfeeding and bedsharing are very interrelated, with a much steeper decline in breastfeeding rates for non-bedsharing babies.[6]

She also noticed that breastfeeding and bedsharing mothers tend to sleep facing their baby in a naturally safe position, with baby's head level with her chest, knees raised to prevent baby slipping under the cover, and an arm bent out around the top of baby's head so baby doesn't creep up the bed; in effect creating a nest for her baby.[7]

However, mothers who have never breastfed and are bedsharing put baby onto a pillow and under bedding. They also turn their back on the baby. They generally sleep with the baby as they would another bed partner.[8]

If you are bottle-feeding, you can still co-sleep. This way you are help-ing your baby bond with you, and fulfilling her need for attachment in other ways. You can also bottle-feed on demand, which is another way of staying in tune with your baby. Try to stick to recommended amounts within a 24-hour period, and go with the flow the rest of the time. There's more on this in the chapter called Sleeping Safely.

I can still remember the desperation we felt on the odd occasions when even breastfeeding didn't work, and our son was incon-solable. The thing that finally worked for us happened almost by accident – I'm addicted to warm baths, and finally just got into a really deep bath and got my husband to hand our baby to me. I put him between my knees and the crying stopped miraculously! The water was up to his chest, and he was able to kick his legs freely.

Whilst we were in hospital, our midwife had told us that a com-mon mistake was to bathe babies in water that was too cold, and so I had made the bath warm enough to be pleasant for me to sit in, and we stayed in there for quite some time, topping up the hot water as required. I always find a hot bath helps with PMT, and can only assume that it helps with colicky tummy aches, too. I also suspect that I probably relaxed somewhat when I got in the bath, and our baby probably responded to that reduction in tension.

After that I gave up on other methods, and just hit the bath whenever the problem arose. We got very accomplished at breast-feeding in the bath, and just put a nice warm towel in the Moses basket next to the bath to wrap him in if he fell asleep. That way I occasionally even had the ultimate luxury of relaxing in the bath alone for five minutes or so!

— *Esther, mother to Rufus*

~ Times Change ~ Answer – 1896 ~

From The Way They Should Go *by Jane Ellen Panton, quoted in*
Christina Hardyment, Dream Babies: Child-care From Locke to Spock
(Jonathan Cape, 1983)

9

Your Baby's Need to Suckle

~ Times change – does the advice stay the same? ~

Trust yourself. You know more than you think you do.

Sucking is pleasurable – even for grown-ups. We chew pencils, suck boiled sweets, smoke cigarettes – none of this is nutritional; we do it because we like the oral stimulation. Why else would we like kissing? One sociobiologist has suggested that kissing is pleasurable because it reminds us of primitive weaning, when mothers used to chew up food for their babies and then spit this puree into the baby's mouth. The flaw in this argument is, of course, that most of us probably have no direct experience of this, our mothers having used tinned food or a food processor! Still, it's an interesting thought to consider next time you are getting intimate with your partner ...

Babies enjoy feeding from breast or bottle not only because it satisfies their hunger and thirst, but also for the oral stimulation.

If you are bottle-feeding, you will be able to see, once the bottle is finished, that your baby has had enough to eat – so what can you do if he still seems to want to suck?

For breastfed babies, you are dependent on cues from your baby to tell when he's had enough to eat, and these are not so easy to spot. Some breastfed babies will get down to business, feed briskly, and then be eager to do other things, but many will linger at the breast, to enjoy the contact. If you are in no hurry, it is fine to let your baby take his time. Sometimes you may be happy to put your feet up and enjoy the closeness. If your baby is unsettled or unwell, allowing him lots of suckling time may be just what is needed, and you can perhaps catch up on some reading, telephone calls or watching some TV. But on other occasions you may want to find different ways for your baby to satisfy his need to suck. The big dilemma is – should you use a dummy?

Dummies – to Suck or Not to Suck?

Everyone has an opinion about dummies! Some think they're fine, others dislike them intensely. Despite strong feelings, there is no strong research evidence to support thumb over dummy or vice versa. What we do know is that anything other than breast in your baby's mouth can cause malocclusion – misalignment of the teeth.[1] Children who use dummies or bottles can grow up to be snorers or have sleep apnoea (where the sufferer briefly stops breathing in their sleep, which is not only disturbing for their partner but is extremely sleep-disrupting).

In addition, using a dummy increases the chance of your baby having middle ear infections by 25 per cent.[2] Dummies also put your baby at greater risk of oral thrush and choking.[3]

There is a growing body of research evidence to suggest that mothers who use dummies may stop breastfeeding earlier than mothers who don't. There are several possible reasons. First, using a dummy means that your baby has less time at the breast and this can affect your milk supply.

Secondly, it may be that the different sucking on a dummy interferes with your baby's learning to suckle on the breast. However, what these studies are

DID YOU KNOW?
One study looked at over 9,000 children aged 3 to 17 and found that those who had been bottle-fed had a 1.84-times higher risk of malocclusion than children who had been breastfed.[4] Another more recent study found that dummies also cause malocclusion, and special physiological or orthodontic dummies make no difference.[5]

not clear about is whether dummies *cause* breastfeeding problems or whether what is happening is that mothers who are having problems with breastfeeding, use dummies.[6]

Is Thumb-sucking Better?

The other problem is that while the research evidence suggests that avoiding dummies might be your safest bet, if your baby wants to suck and you don't give him a dummy or allow him to spend as long as he wants on the breast, he may well opt for his thumb instead. In fact, babies are born with the ability to soothe themselves: the Babkin reflex ensures that baby will put his hand to his mouth to suck if he wants this kind of comfort. However, this reflex is lost at around five to six weeks old, which is perhaps why crying peaks at this age.[7] If you introduce a dummy at this time instead, he may never use his fingers.[8]

While orthodontists frown upon long-term dummy-sucking, they think long-term thumb-sucking is equally bad.[9] Speech therapists also believe extensive sucking on either dummy or thumb is a bad idea, as both may change the structure of the mouth and cause speech problems later on.

What the research on malocclusion does indicate is that the problems are made worse if your baby sucks several times during the day, for long stretches, and if he carries on with it for several months. Therefore, if you want to strike a balance between possible harm and soothing your baby, you might be better using a dummy in moderation, while also allowing your baby to have plenty of time at the breast, and using other methods of soothing, too. It would also probably be sensible not to allow the dummy to become associated with falling asleep (see the section on Step Three for more about this). In addition:

- **Try to get rid of the dummy before it becomes an attachment object; at around six months perhaps.**
- **Never pin it to his clothes with string, as this can be a choking hazard.**

DID YOU KNOW?
One interesting piece of research looked at how to soothe babies who were undergoing unpleasant medical procedures. They found that the most effective form of pain-relief other than drugs was sucking on a dummy, which was more effective than concentrated sucrose and glucose, or no treatment at all. However, using sucrose *and* a dummy was the most effective analgesic of all,[10] which is probably why people used to dip dummies in honey. However, honey is **not** recommended for infants, as it can give babies botulism, and sucking on a sweetened dummy is extremely bad for your baby's developing teeth.

GETTING YOUR BABY TO TAKE A DUMMY

If your baby spits out his dummy, try offering it to him when he's calm, and the minute he starts to suck on it even lightly, tug it as if you were going to take it away. This will make him grip it a little harder, and if you keep tugging it gently, he will eventually suck it firmly.

Getting a breastfed baby to take a dummy can be difficult, as the first thing a breastfed baby does when offered something to suck, is to thrust out his tongue, and if they do that with a dummy it gets dislodged. One suggestion is to try gently holding the dummy in place for a count of eight to start with. If it comes back out after that, then he probably doesn't want it.[11]

THUMB/FINGERS – ADVANTAGES

- **Your baby is in control. He can find his own thumb when he's miserable, or if he wakes in the night, rather than needing you.**
- **No need to sterilize and no worry about losing it.**

THUMB/FINGERS – DISADVANTAGES

- **Can be harder to stop the habit.**
- **As you cannot control how much or how often he sucks, he may be at risk of distorting his developing mouth, so he may need lots of expensive and difficult orthodontic work later.**

DUMMY – ADVANTAGES

- **You can get rid of it more easily than thumb sucking.**
- **You can use it for a fretful baby before he is capable of finding his thumb.**

DUMMY – DISADVANTAGES

- **Health hazards – every time it drops you need to sterilize it.**
- **If he becomes attached to it for sleeping, you will need to find it for him in the night.**

One morning it was so quiet I went in to see what she was up to. She had managed to find BOTH her thumbs, and she was sucking on them vigorously with her legs sticking straight up in the air with pleasure!

– Belinda, mother to Poppy

~ Times Change ~ Answer – 1955 ~

From Baby and Child Care *by Dr Benjamin Spock*

STEP TWO

Comfort

10

Recreating the Womb

~ Times change – does the advice stay the same? ~

*There was something so natural as well as pleasant in the wavy
motion of the cradle ... and so like what children had been used
to before they were born.*

There is no doubt that human beings give birth to the most
dependent babies on the planet. Some mammals are able to walk
almost immediately, and even our nearest relatives, the apes, are
capable of supporting their own heads and clinging onto their
mothers' fur.

Some writers have suggested that all human babies are born 'premature'; that babies have to be born before their heads get too big to fit
through the pelvis, which means they arrive before they are really
ready to support themselves, and they need another three months in
the womb.[1]

An interesting theory, but of course babies are born capable of many things – they have excellent control over their facial muscles, allowing them to communicate subtly with whoever is looking after them, as well as allowing them to take milk actively from their mother's breasts. They can vocalize to the extent of being able to cry. Human babies may not survive on their own, but they have all these wonderful tools at their disposal to make sure they don't have to – they can depend on us grown-ups.

Whether or not they actually need more time in the womb, babies do seem to enjoy sensations which remind them of being in the womb, perhaps because these are familiar and evoke pleasant memories. You can use these associations to calm your fretful baby.

What's It Like for Your Baby in the Womb? – The Five 'Senses'

1 **Smell**. Believe it or not, foetuses can smell! Scents carry in amniotic fluid, and your baby's sense of smell develops at around 28 weeks' gestation. Throughout the third trimester, she can smell everything her Mum can, as the placenta becomes more permeable, allowing in molecules from the outside world. This is probably why a newborn baby can identify her Mum after

There is also evidence that unwashed babies are more successful at bringing their hands to their mouths to self-comfort in the first hour after birth. Within six days, your baby will recognize the smell of your milk. Older babies are thought to scent-mark their parents with their saliva – through breastfeeding and, later, through tears and general drool! This is also how attachment objects (cuddlies) become important, and why children get so upset if a favourite teddy is washed.[2]

birth; research has shown that newborns respond to the smell of their own amniotic fluid, and prefer to feed from a breast moistened with amniotic fluid.[3]

2 **Vision**. Light comes and goes inside the womb, but it's never bright. Sometimes there's a dim red glow, as light shines through mother's skin and blood vessels, but if Mum is wearing clothes it may be completely dark, as it is at night. The sense of sight is not important in the womb, and after your baby is born she may not rely on sight as much as her other senses, although some babies are more 'visual' than others. Babies can see straight after birth, but it will be like looking through opaque glass – hard to focus on anything but strong contrasts. The range of their focus is about 8 to 12 inches.

3 **Movement**. At times, she will be jiggled around as her mother gets on with her daily activities. When this happens she may lie still to experience the wonderful rocking and swaying sensations. When her mother rests or sleeps, the motion stops, and often she will kick and squirm to recreate these sensations. The vestibular system, which is responsible for our sense of motion and balance, and is located in the ear, is one of our most primitive and therefore one of the earliest to emerge in your baby's development, and is the next to develop after touch. It is responsible for the Moro or startle reflex, among others.[4]

4 **Touch**. All around, the temperature is constant and really warm. She feels herself tightly held by the uterine muscles, but also there's a feeling of weightlessness, as she's suspended in amniotic fluid – a bit like floating in a deep warm pool. Premature babies as young as 25 weeks' gestation are aware of touch, and this seems to be the earliest sensation your baby will recognize. Touch develops from head to toe – so the mouth is the first region to become sensitive – which is why young babies and children put everything in their mouths.[5]

5 **Sound**. Interestingly, it is now thought that hearing is the most important sense for the foetus, providing a connection with the outside world. There is constant noise – the booming sound of Mum's heart and gurgling and whooshing noises from her digestion. Sound levels vary between 30 and 96 decibels, depending on what Mum is doing.[7]
Lower frequency actually penetrates better than higher, so Dad's voice travels well, though Mum's is clearest as it's coming directly through her body.

> **DID YOU KNOW?**
> **– Touch is the most important sense for your baby.**
> In one experiment, babies were given different shaped dummies to suck on without seeing them. When they were shown larger versions of these later on, they were able to identify the dummies they had sucked on before.[6]

Researchers have found that babies in the womb respond to music, particularly Mum singing. They seem to dislike rock, opera and jazz, although there are always exceptions! Foetuses also begin to tune in to the language they will speak, so that from birth they move their bodies in synchrony to human speech – and research has shown that they do it better for their own tongue than for a foreign language.[8]

Creating Another Womb for Your Baby

In the early months of your baby's life, you can use the knowledge of what the womb felt like to comfort and soothe her. We will look at using sound, touch and movement in the next two chapters; for now, let's concentrate on sight and smell.

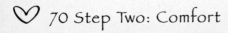

Being aware that your baby's vision is blurry can help if she is fretting when you can see her, as it may well be that she can't see you! Her eyes focus best at approximately 8 to 12 inches.

Smell is a much stronger sense for her, which might be difficult to replicate but it is useful to be aware of just how strong your baby's sense of smell is early on, and perhaps to avoid using strong perfumes or detergents. Contact is more important though, to allow her to get to know your smell in the first place. We know this because breastfed babies can identify their own mother's smell at birth, but bottle-fed babies cannot recognize their own mother's smell at two weeks, and neither breast nor bottle-fed babies recognize their father's scent. However you are feeding your baby, if you hold her so that her skin is next to your skin, you will be helping her to bond with you.

Some of the tools at your disposal will work really well, but your baby might be indifferent to others. What works today might not work tomorrow. That's fine – your baby is her own character and, as you are finding out, she has her own definite opinions! Just a couple of points, though:

- It's best to try only one strategy at a time. This helps you spot what's working.
- Give her time to register what you are doing and respond. Think about how long it takes her to smile back at you or imitate you sticking out your tongue, even when she's paying attention.

Will My Baby Grow to Depend on These Soothing Strategies?

As your baby grows and develops, these womb strategies will probably become less effective as she accumulates pleasant memories of experiences of life outside the womb. However, some of them may remain as a comfort in stressful times, and that's perfectly normal. Adults, too, in times of emotional distress will want to be held and hugged for comfort. But don't worry; it's extremely unlikely that your children will grow up into teenagers who prefer to listen to the Hoover or washing machine!

DID YOU KNOW?
– The womb works!
One study compared infants sleeping in a normal cot, with those sleeping in a cot specifically designed to feel similar to the womb; it moved, had sound and held the babies firmly. The babies with the special cribs cried significantly less during the study period, slept for longer periods at night and slept through the night sooner.[11]

I sat at 3 a.m. on the floor with my little one cradled in one arm and the hairdryer on at full pelt in the other. For some strange reason it stopped the crying. Mad moments like this kept my sanity.

— *Iona, mother to Sebastian and Francesca*

~ Times Change ~ Answer – 1789 ~

From Michael Underwood, Treatise on the Diseases of Children, *quoted in Dr Harvey Karp,* The Happiest Baby on the Block *(Penguin/Michael Joseph, 2002)*

11

Using Sound and Movement

~ **Times change – does the advice stay the same?** ~
*When a baby wakes out of a long deep sleep he should be ready to
laugh. But if he has been disturbed, he will be fretful. This is a
reflex from the vague feeling of misery caused by the incomplete
natural cleansing of all the dirt accumulation of his system.*

Where there is a need, there is a market, and you can now buy 'womb
noise' tapes as well as womb-noise teddies! Be assured that in fact
the sound of a tumble dryer, extractor fan, running water, vacuum
cleaner or hairdryer work just as well, as does playing the radio when
it is not tuned to any station, so you hear the static or 'white noise'.
You can experiment and perhaps tape the sound your baby seems to
like best.

If the idea of playing white noise to your baby drives you mad, why
not play something that appeals to your own taste? Many babies love
music, and they can be quite selective in their choice! If classical is

not to his liking, try rock and roll, and if you dance along with your baby in your arms, he'll have double the pleasure! We know that babies remember the music they hear during pregnancy; so if you had a favourite tune you listened to when you were pregnant, why not try it out again now?[1]

If your baby is not one for loud music, try singing lullabies to him. He will probably particularly like it if you hum or sing softly while resting your head against his. The word lullaby means 'to sing to sleep',[2] and it is interesting to think about how many lullabies have a rhythm which coincides with our own heartbeat! Clever!

The shh sound is the root of the word asking for silence in many languages, and if you say it loudly enough, it acts like your own, portable, white noise tape. Shhh![3]

Comforting Your Baby with Movement

Babies love to be in motion, and the more vigorous the better. You can dance with your baby, jiggling round the room in time to your favourite music; you can take him for car rides, perhaps en route to see other new mums in a postnatal support group, or to have a good walk in the country with your baby in a sling, back-pack or pushchair.

Walking out with your baby every day is such a good idea:

DID YOU KNOW? – Womb noise works!
One midwife found that a womb noise tape was effective 98.4 per cent of the time in soothing the babies in her care, and when it wasn't, the baby was due for a feed. She went on to contrast this with taped lullabies, and found it took fewer than 5 minutes to calm a baby with womb noise, compared to an average 10 minutes without.[4]

it's healthy exercise, you both get lots of fresh air, and getting out of the house will help you avoid developing postnatal depression.

Some newborn babies have times when they feel 'disorganized' – flailing about and showing body tension as well as crying. Babies who are held and carried feel more organized, as well as showing greater visual alertness than those comforted in other ways. In fact, it is during these times of quiet alertness that babies can most effectively absorb information about the world around them.[5]

If your baby wants to be held or jigged around a lot of the time, get other people to hold him, too; he won't mind who is doing the carrying. Invest in a good sling; the ones with lots of different positions will probably last you longer, but ask around for recommendations and borrow a few to try out. Some slings don't have enough support so your baby outgrows them very quickly.

Don't ever try jigging or bouncing with your baby if you are angry or really upset – not only will you communicate these emotions to him, making him more upset, but you could just be in danger of shaking him too hard.

You don't have to carry your baby all the time unless you want to; you can buy a fancy chair that will do all the rocking for you, and it will even match your womb conditions precisely. In the womb, he was probably rocked forwards and backwards, rather than side to side, and researchers have found that this is how babies like to be rocked, with the most effective at comforting your baby corresponding to that produced by your pelvis as you walk, a maximum of 60 rocks per minute swinging 2¾ inches.[6] (Can't you just picture researchers in white coats with clipboards testing this out on a roomful of crying babies?)

My first baby was due at around Christmas, and I listened to Handel's *Messiah* in the car on the way to work. After he was born, one particularly miserable morning I decided to try to drown out his crying with a few Hallelujahs from Handel – and was amazed when he instantly stopped crying; listening instead with an expression of rapture on his face!

– Caroline, mother of Alasdair, Chris and Josie
(and author of the book!)

~ Times Change ~ Answer – 1939 ~
From Marie Stopes, Your Baby's First Year, *quoted in Christina Hardyment,*
Dream Babies: Child-care From Locke to Spock *(Jonathan Cape, 1983)*

12

The Power of Touch

~ **Times change – does the advice stay the same?** ~
*Babies less than six months old should never be played with
at all. To avoid over-stimulation, babies need peaceful and
quiet surroundings.*

Do you know which is the biggest organ in the human body? It's your
skin. Laid flat, it would cover an area of about 21 square feet. It pro-
tects us, and is the means through which we experience one of our most
profound and important senses. We can live a life without sight or
sound, but not without touch. Babies born without effective nerve con-
nections between skin and brain can fail to thrive and can even die.[1]

'In touching cultures, adult aggression is low, whereas in cultures
where touch is limited, adult aggression is high,' claims Tiffany Field,
director of the Touch Research Institutes at the University of Miami
School of Medicine.[2]

The Earliest Touch – Inside the Womb

As we have seen, your baby is used to being held tightly, unable to move inside the womb. You can recreate the feeling of restricted space by wrapping your baby firmly in a cot blanket. Many babies love to be wrapped ('swaddled'), others resist it, but if you persevere you may find she will settle once she's swaddled. Sometimes swaddling is useful to keep your baby from flailing about so that you can get through to her with other calming methods. Swaddling is also great for the baby whose little fingers always seem to be in the way when you're trying to latch her on for a breastfeed! (Don't wrap up her hands too often, though, as babies need to be able to use their hands and fingers, their earliest tools.)

Swaddling has been found not only to pacify babies, it also helps them to sleep. Swaddled babies spend more time asleep even if they're only swaddled above the waist, and perhaps because they are easier to handle when they are trussed up, swaddled infants tend to spend more time in physical and social contact with adults.[3]

Swaddling goes back at least to Roman times, but some time in the 18th century it became unfashionable in England, and died out.[4] Despite what you might think, swaddled babies develop perfectly normally – Hopi Indian babies spend much of their first year strapped to a cradleboard on their mother's back, and yet they begin walking at around 15 months, which is within the normal range.[5]

HOW TO 'SWADDLE' A BABY

Place a large cot blanket on the floor, and lay it in a diamond shape, folding the top point over to create a flat edge for your baby's shoulders to lie along. Bring one top corner across to tuck under her bottom, and bring the bottom point up to tuck into this wrap. You can wrap the other top corner around her and tuck the corner in to secure in the material at her neck. She is now firmly contained.

Warmth

The other sensation from being in the womb was, of course, being immersed in warm water. Even as adults we love that feeling – just think how relaxing a really hot, deep bath feels! Many babies love being bathed for that reason, but others seem to panic – why? Probably because of the way we lower them into the bath.

MAKING BATHS LESS SCARY

One of the most disconcerting experiences for a helpless baby is to feel she's falling or being dropped, and babies have an emergency reflex – the Moro reflex – where they fling out their arms in a last-ditch attempt to prevent themselves being hurt. So if your baby panics about the bath, just 'top and tail' her (your midwife will show you how) or try bathing her tummy-down, making sure you keep one hand under her chin to keep her face clear of the water or, better still, get into the bath with her and let her lie on your tummy in the water.

This is an excellent way, too, of getting a baby to latch onto the breast when all else seems to be failing. You will probably need help to get out of the bath afterwards, so don't attempt this when you are alone in the house!

What You Can Do

SKIN TO SKIN

Holding your naked baby next to your naked body is soothing for both of you. It is also useful to breastfeed your baby skin-to-skin if she is finding latching on difficult. One study compared newborn babies who received skin-to-skin contact with a group who were kept next to their mother in a cot. The skin-to-skin newborns cried less and had increased body temperatures and blood sugar levels.[7]

MASSAGE

Your baby may also find a massage soothing. You don't need to be an expert – watch your baby for clues as to what she likes. Use slow, stroking movements, keeping one hand in contact with her body at all times. You don't need to use any oil, but if you find it helpful, then a vegetable oil is probably safest. You cannot use aromatherapy oils or scents, as these are too strong for babies.

Research suggests that premature babies gain more weight, go home from hospital earlier, and are less likely to have postnatal complications, if they are massaged,[8] and in one study, pre-term babies who had been massaged performed better in IQ tests at age six months than those who had not been massaged.[9] Massage was also found to be effective in reducing the amount of time a colicky baby cried.[10]

> **DID YOU KNOW?**
> **– Touch makes you brainier!**
> Researchers have found that if young rats are given lots of different toys to touch, their somatosensory cortexes – the part of the brain responsible for experiencing touch – gets bigger, but if the same toys are left in their cage, the rats grow bored with them and their cortexes begin to shrink back in size. This doesn't mean you need to buy hundreds of different cuddly toys, though – the same thing happened if the rat mums gave them extra grooming, or if the experimenters handled them more in their early weeks of life.[6]

If you find you and your baby enjoy massage, then you might like to go to special classes where parents are taught to massage their children. Contacts are given in the Useful Organizations and Further Reading chapter.

I first used massage to ease my baby's colic, and I now teach baby massage to small groups of mums, for colic and for general relaxation of their babies. It usually soothes the mums, too. I try to get the mothers to feel calm and relaxed themselves before we give the massage, as babies seem to pick up on their mothers' mood! Calm Mum – calm baby. Tense Mum – tense baby.

– Jean, mother of Laura

~ Times Change ~ Answer – early 1900s ~

From Dr Emett Holt, Care and Feeding of Children

13

Comforting the Baby Who Has Colic

~ Times change – does the advice stay the same? ~

It is with great pleasure I see at last the preservation of children become the care of Men of Sense. This business has been too long fatally left to the management of women, who cannot be supposed to have a proper knowledge to fit them for the task.

It's not supposed to be like this – having a baby that cries for hours on end as if in pain. Everything you try works for a couple of minutes, and then he's off again. You were expecting a smiling, contented tot, but instead your baby is thoroughly miserable. People say 'Oh, it's colic; it will pass,' but your need is to do something for your baby right now.

There is little agreement among professionals about what causes colic, but all parents who have experienced it can describe it: Your baby seems inconsolable, and cries for what feels like hours on end.

Colic usually affects babies at around two weeks of age, peaks at around six weeks, and tails off after the third month. Some babies cry on and off for much of the day, but mostly colic hits in the evenings, with some continuing to cry long past any reasonably civilized bed-time. Many parents report their baby drawing his legs up as if he were experiencing cramps or tummy ache. Their baby desperately wants to suck, but even when he has fed, he is still unhappy.

When colic affects your baby, it can feel as if your world has been turned upside down. You so enjoyed becoming a parent, but now you have this miserable baby to deal with – this is not what you expected. No one seems to understand or want to help; perhaps your GP and your health visitor shrug it off as a 'phase', or perhaps their advice doesn't seem to work. It is understandable if you feel depressed, even angry.

Definition of Colic

Researchers had, at least for a while, agreed on a definition, what was called Wessel's Rule of Threes: your baby has colic if he cries at least three hours a

**DID YOU KNOW?
– You need understanding!**
One researcher for a health visitors' journal carried out in-depth interviews with 14 families in West Yorkshire, to suggest ways health professionals could help families with babies with colic. What he found was that parents of babies with colic had four specific needs:

1. for people to listen and try to understand
2. to be believed
3. for someone to visit and to be there
4. for reassurance that the parents are not to blame and that the crying will stop.

Many of the parents he spoke to felt professionals had not believed them, and that generally people did not try to understand their problem.[1]

day, on more than three days in one week.[2] This has now been modified, as it has been recognized that if your baby cries for two and a half hours a day, it may still feel like a lot! Most researchers now focus on lots of crying and/or fussing, which is intense and almost impossible to soothe.[3]

What they haven't agreed about is the cause. Although there has been quite a lot of research in the area, nothing conclusive has been discovered. The truth is probably that there are lots of different reasons for a baby to cry for long periods of time, and you will need to consider all of them to work out how to help your baby.

Is It Just a Sore Tummy?

The word *colic* derives from the Greek word 'kolikos', meaning large intestine or colon, and as such seems to imply that it is about indigestion or stomach pain, but when researchers put tape-recorders in the homes of colicky babies, although they could indeed record the amount babies cried and agreed that it was excessive, the nature of the crying wasn't substantially different to the cries of babies who were known not to be in pain,[4] although as we have seen earlier in this book, pain cries are not necessarily easy to identify.

Parents usually believe that their colicky baby is in pain; first because he seems inconsolable, and secondly because he often draws his knees up as if he has wind or stomach cramps. However, another study using x-rays did not often reveal anything particularly different about the tummies of most colicky babies.[5] The problem is that when a baby is upset and crying vigorously, he may well draw his knees up – he will cry with his entire being! So, while it is worth exploring factors which might cause your baby to have tummy trouble, do remember that having colic doesn't necessarily mean your baby has a sore tummy.

In fact, for this reason, colic is now more often referred to as 'unexplained crying', where babies cry for *longer* than average, are harder to *console*, and their cries are generally *louder* and tend to be at a *particular time of day.*

If you think your baby is in pain, you should consult your doctor in case there is a more serious problem. This is particularly true if he cries all day, if crying continues after four months, or if your baby has any other symptoms like fever, sickness, tummy upset or weight loss.

Does Crying Have Any Benefits?

It may help a little if you can see that there are some benefits to your baby of crying! Crying actually evolved in mammals as part of 'homeothermy', which means maintaining a stable body temperature. Experiments with baby rats show that even when they are so cold that they are hypothermic and in a coma, they will still cry, but once they start to warm up due to contact with their mothers, they stop crying. Crying actually raises their body temperatures and helps prevent pulmonary oedema, a side-effect of going from being excessively cold to being at normal temperature again.[6]

Crying also triggers 'the let-down reflex' in mammal mothers; where milk is squeezed down from high in the breast to the nipple where the baby can get it. Breastfeeding mothers may find that milk leaks when they hear a baby's cry, and most mothers will try feeding a crying baby as a first strategy. Colicky babies rarely fail to thrive, while babies who do fail to thrive are often those who sleep through the night early and don't cry much.

Of course, over the millions of years of our evolution food shortages were perhaps the biggest threat to survival, so a baby who cried loudly and got fed was more likely to survive. Loud and persistent crying makes perfect evolutionary sense; the problem is that we now live in a culture where food is plentiful and there is no need to cry lustily to ensure you get the most – but our babies haven't cottoned onto that fact yet!

The third and final function of excessive crying might be that good old-fashioned idea – exercise! Crying stimulates the organization of the vocal respiratory apparatus which we humans use in talking. So, some unexplained early crying might be for exercise, and that might be another reason why carrying is so effective in reducing crying. If babies are carried by their mothers, they are being stimulated, reducing the need to cry, but if they're motionlesss they cry as a form of self-stimulation.[7]

Coping with Colic

A baby who cannot be comforted is devastating. When your baby is crying, it's all too easy to get wound up yourself. However, you need to stay calm if at all possible, as your baby will sense your tension and this can make things worse. It can help to realize that many babies go through this, and your aim is to let your baby know you are there for him, but not get drawn into his anxiety.

It is worth remembering, perhaps, that although your baby may seem upset for many hours, he will not actually remember this when he's older, and if his experience of you is as someone caring and consistent, the fact that he had times when he cried will not be as emotionally damaging as you might think.

SHARE THE BURDEN
Make sure your family, friends and your partner take turns comforting him; your baby won't mind at this stage who is doing the cuddling. It can also be a great help to meet up with other new mums

with colicky babies; ask your local NCT or health visitor to put you in touch. If you feel you are losing your temper, then put your baby in his cot and walk away until you calm down; ring someone to talk things over.

- **Get help from your family, your friends and your partner. No one should have to cope with a colicky baby alone.**
- **Try one strategy at a time. This way you might be clearer about what is working and what is not.**
- **Always eliminate all physical possibilities first if you can, no matter how remote these may seem, especially if the crying is all day, and/or if it goes on beyond three months.**
- **It is worth keeping a diary of your baby's crying and fussing behaviour. You may be able to identify particular triggers this way, and it will also be useful if you seek medical help at a later time.**

Our baby cried a lot when he was born, but was soothed when I sang him the song I'd sung in the last two months of pregnancy whenever I was relaxing or quietly doing something. It seemed to still him and help him to relax. In the evenings, at the worst colicky time, we really only helped him by walking up and down the stairs with him. He used to lie face-down on my husband's forearm, facing towards his elbow, so that Freddie's hand was supporting his stomach. I imagined that the warmth from the hand and the gentle movement were helpful to him. One night when he was very small and couldn't stop crying I was at my wit's end and decided to give him a bath ... at 2 a.m.! It worked!

*– Nicola, **mother of Alistair.***

~ Times Change ~ Answer – 1748 ~

From William Cadogan, Essay on Nursing *in Christina Hardyment,*
Dream Babies: Child-care From Locke to Spock *(Jonathan Cape, 1983)*

14

Feeding the Baby with Colic

~ Times change – does the advice stay the same? ~

I would make it a criminal offence for mothers to attempt to impose their personality on their children. Certain things have been proved to be of use in this world, and these things can best be taught by men. You can't get them from the average mother – they aren't in her.

It is really tempting to think that what you are feeding your baby is probably the root of the colic problem. However, whether your baby is fed breastmilk or formula milk may not make as much difference to colic as you might think.

Why Does My Baby Want to Feed So Often?

The colicky baby may or may not be hungry, but as sucking is the best comfort she knows, she will want to return to the breast or bottle as often as she can. Sucking helps her move gas along her intestine; this is why your baby may have loud wind while she's feeding!

It's really easy to worry about her appetite – this is part of being a parent, and won't go away even when she's older! Try to remember that a baby who is genuinely starving will become quiet and passive, whimpering rather than bawling healthily.

Is She Constipated?

If you are breastfeeding, it is unlikely your baby will get constipated. Some babies, particularly in the early days, don't like the sensation of having a bowel motion and may cry while they do, but even if she does seem to strain, don't worry if the result is still soft – normally yellow and the consistency of scrambled eggs. Perhaps she looks under strain because the sensation is new to her; after all, it must feel weird the first few times!

Bottle-fed babies can get constipated, so if she's having problems, discuss with your health visitor the possibility of changing formula, as some seem to agree with babies better than others.

DID YOU KNOW?
– Breastfed babies have similar levels of colic to formula fed babies.
The only real difference that has been found is in the pattern of crying. One longitudinal study compared breastfed babies with formula-fed babies, and found that while breastfed babies' crying peaked at six weeks, formula-fed babies' crying peaked earlier, at two weeks. The intense crying/colic behaviour occurred in 43 per cent of formula-fed babies and just 16 per cent of those fed by breast.[1]

Winding Your Baby

If your baby seems to need to bring up wind:

- **Sit her upright on your lap with your hand under her chin, keeping her back as straight as possible. Your baby will probably be leaning forward slightly. Then you can pat her back quite firmly.**

Alternatively:

- **First put a good absorbent towel over your shoulder reaching well down your back.**
- **Prop her over your shoulder, so she's upright, her chin resting on your shoulder and her tummy stretched out full-length against your chest.**
- **Stroke her back and sides firmly and slowly upwards towards her neck several times. Quite firm pressure is needed, like stroking a cat really hard, backwards!**

Help for Colicky Bottle-fed Babies

Some parents find using different types of bottle or teat can work. If baby is windy, you could try a teat which slows down the milk flow. You could also feed your baby in a more upright position, with frequent pauses to allow trapped air to escape. Feeding little and often seems to help some bottle-fed colicky babies.

If cow's milk intolerance is suspected, your doctor or health visitor might suggest using hypoallergenic formula milk, only available on prescription. Formula milk based on soya is less effective in treating colic, and is high in phytoestrogens, to the extent that a diet of exclusively soya-based baby milk is equivalent to consuming several contraceptive pills every day.[2] In any case, it's best not to swap brands or types of formula without consulting your health visitor.

Breastfeeding and Colic

Many mothers wonder if their baby is reacting to something in their breastmilk. This is possible, but hard to pinpoint, as you need to exclude items from your diet for up to two weeks to see any difference, and then 'challenge' the baby by reintroducing various products in your diet, one by one, to see if symptoms recur.[3]

The most common triggers are:

- **Cow's milk proteins. If you or your partner have a family history of allergies – for instance, eczema or asthma, coeliac disease or other food intolerance, then it is worth considering this, especially if your baby has been given a 'top up' of formula at some point which could have sensitized her. Excluding dairy produce from your diet is difficult, and you need to ensure that you have alternative forms of calcium – see the appendix (page 183) for a cow's milk-free diet.**
- **Caffeine – found in tea, coffee, cola and chocolate – although most babies can cope with moderate amounts.**
- **One very small pilot study suggested that zinc supplements in breastfeeding mothers might reduce colicky crying.[4] The numbers in the study were so small no firm conclusions could be drawn, but many people do have a shortage of zinc in their diet, and as supplementing your diet with zinc will do no harm and may do you some good, it could be worth trying.**
- **Some cruciferous vegetables have also been related to colic symptoms; namely cabbage, cauliflower, broccoli and onions.[5]**

It is estimated that up to 25 per cent of colicky babies[6] have a problem digesting cow's milk proteins,[7] so it is certainly worth discussing this with a health professional. The normal treatment for this would be to exclude cow's milk proteins from the baby's diet for at least two weeks to see if there is any improvement, and then 'challenge' the baby by reintroducing it to see if symptoms recur.

Lactose Intolerance

This life-threatening but rare disorder takes the form of an allergy-like reaction to *lactose*, the sugar in all mammal milks, including human milk. The level of lactose in breastmilk is at a constant level and has nothing to do with whether you're eating dairy products. Foremilk does not contain more lactose, though it does contain less fat – see below.

Lactose intolerance occurs when someone does not have enough of the enzyme *lactase* to digest lactose. Nearly all babies produce enough lactase; levels start to fall from about three to five years of age, when they would naturally wean from the breast. Lactose intolerance is extremely rare in babies – and a baby with lactose intolerance would fail to thrive from birth.[8]

In cultures where cow's milk is consumed by adults (mostly those of Northern European descent), lactase tends to continue to be produced throughout life, but 70 per cent of the world's population have such low levels of lactase that they are lactose intolerant as adults – mostly in races such as Asian, African, Australian Aboriginal and Hispanic. It is worth remembering that even babies born into these races can digest lactose without difficulty.

LACTOSE OVERLOAD

Lactose overload can look like lactose intolerance, but is to do with how a baby feeds, not a lack of lactase.

At the beginning of a breastfeed, the milk your baby drinks is called *foremilk*, which is low in fat. As the feed progresses, this gradually changes into *hindmilk*, which contains the same amount of lactose but has more fat. If your baby's feed is mostly foremilk, it will pass through her system so quickly that not all the lactose is digested. When it reaches her lower bowel, it draws in extra water and ferments, producing gas, acidy stools and tummy pain.[9] The surest sign of lactose overload is a baby who is unsettled even after feeding, and who has green, explosive nappies.

You could imagine how it feels by thinking of a diet of lemonade. Although you would seem full initially, you would start to feel uncomfortable, a bit gassy, and you would soon be hungry again.

To ensure that your baby is getting enough hindmilk, it is worth asking a breastfeeding counsellor to check your baby's positioning. Often, just a slight change can make all the difference.

It is also generally good practice to let baby decide when she's had enough rather than trying to limit her time at the breast. If, however, your baby is snacking little and often, she may be getting more foremilk, so you might like to think about allocating one breast for a certain period of time, and every time within that period your baby wants to feed, put her back to the same breast, rather than swapping breasts too often.

Research has found that prolonged feeding on one breast, offering the second breast only if the baby still seems hungry, leads to less colic than when women feed from both breasts equally at each feed.[10] However, it should also be said that the best way to feed your baby is to let her decide when she's had enough, which she will indicate by coming off the breast, and then it is best practice to offer the other breast as well.

Usually a breastfed baby can regulate her own fat intake, and your milk supply would normally adjust to meet her needs, so try not to get too hung up about one breast, two breasts – follow the pattern that seems to suit your baby and it will usually be fine.[11]

The other issue is that the more your baby stimulates your breasts, the more milk you will produce, and if you have a large supply, it will mean, of course, that your baby will have more foremilk to drink before the hindmilk comes through. Ironically, many mothers start to believe that they don't have enough milk if their baby wants to feed all the time, when in fact what they have is a bit of an over-supply problem.

TOO MUCH MILK?

If you have an oversupply problem, then your baby will also be unsettled and feeding a lot, but will probably have good weight gain and lots of messy nappies. Again, a breastfeeding counsellor can help; you could also think about designating one breast for a time period, as before, to reduce stimulation on your breasts and ease your supply down – though be careful you don't let your breasts get too full when you're doing this.

You could also try to space feeds out a bit more, if you can. It might be that if baby wants to suck you could let her suck on your finger, or you could try a dummy – have a look at page 60 for more on this.

My son Jake didn't have an ounce of colic, so I was dismayed when Beth started to show signs of being colicky in her second week. To start with we did all the usual – pacing the floor and whatnot – but two things really helped: sticking our finger in her mouth to give her something to suck, and seeing a breastfeeding counsellor.

Everything I read about colic seemed to point to the fact that colic can be caused by a bad latch. I had breastfed Jake for 15 months, so thought I could do latches, but it still nagged at me. And the breastfeeding counsellor I saw when Beth was about three or four weeks agreed that our latch wasn't great, and put us straight. That evening the colic disappeared, and by working really hard on our new positioning, the colic had gone altogether by the time she was six weeks old.

– Kedi, mum to Jake and Beth

~ Times Change ~ Answer – 1911 ~

John Masefield, 'The street today', in Christina Hardyment,
Dream Babies: Child-care From Locke to Spock (*Jonathan Cape, 1983*)

15

Is Your Colicky Baby Oversensitive?

~ Times change – does the advice stay the same? ~

A hundred years ago it was rare not to feed one's baby oneself.
Now custom has changed this; the query, 'how do you feed him?'
is conventional.

Despite what you might have been told, colic is not your fault! Research used to concentrate on the mother – her personality, whether she was depressed and so on - but no one really found anything significant about the mothers of crying babies, although researchers did find that the mother of a baby who cries excessively can become depressed or lose confidence – not surprising, really.[1]

You might find yourself beginning to think that your baby is crying deliberately, especially if well-meaning (but misguided) outsiders say things like 'You're spoiling him.' Do remember that at this age your baby is incapable of manipulative behaviour; all he knows is that he has a need, and you are the only person who can try to sort it out for him. As he gets older, he will learn other ways of communicating his needs, but for now crying is his only option.

Is Colic a Normal Part of Your Baby's Development?

Recent research has focused on the idea that excessive crying or colic is developmental, and therefore outside parental control. For instance, for premature babies colic starts later, so it happens at around the time they would have been six weeks old if they had been born at their due date.[2]

Linked to this is the theory that colicky crying is a bit like 'jet lag': your baby is reorganizing his internal workings to cope with a day/night cycle. Another theory claims that the crying is delayed shock from birth. Still other people suggest that having too much information to process causes the fretfulness – this is why it occurs in the evening. By the time your baby gets to 6 o'clock, his brain has become overloaded, but can't shut down.

The point to stress here is that most forms of colic are developmental and *neurological* – arising from the brain – rather than *digestive*. If you look at it this way, for most crying babies colic is something they *do* rather than a condition they *have*. This is supported by evidence that, although in different societies the average amount of time babies cry varies, there is still a developmental pattern of crying increasing after the first few weeks of life, reaching a peak and then decreasing several weeks later.[3]

Overtired?

Babies are not born with the ability to fall asleep easily; this is something we have to learn, as we will see. In fact, adults have similar problems – if we've been terribly busy all day, we can find it hard to get to sleep even though we're desperately tired.

Your baby has to cope with so many new sights and sounds during the course of a routine day; perhaps it feels impossible for him to be calm in the evenings. As many babies have a developmental growth spurt at around two weeks, six weeks and again at three months, these are common times for him to feel particularly mentally over-stretched.

If you think this applies to your baby, then try creating a structured, early bedtime, perhaps with a soothing bath, a gentle cuddle and last feed *before* the miserable time starts. You can also cut down on stimulating events late afternoon, and have a look at the section on sleep.

A Stressful Start to Life?

There is some evidence that mothers who were doing shift-work during pregnancy were more likely to report colicky crying, while mothers who had a partner and full-time employment while pregnant, were less likely to have a baby who cried excessively.[4]

Another large-scale study in Finland found an association between stress in pregnancy or negative experiences during childbirth and colic.[5] What on earth can this mean? Well, what it could mean is that one cause of colic could be stress during pregnancy. Sheila Kitzinger found, when researching her book *The Crying Baby*, that 60 per cent of the women she talked to whose babies cried excessively (and by this she meant more than six hours in 24) had had a stressful pregnancy. Perhaps some babies, whose passage into the world was difficult, have a difficult time adjusting to life.

One large study of over 2,000 babies in Denmark found that low-weight babies were more likely to have colic according to the Wessel definitions.[6] While most pre-term babies don't cry more than full-term babies, there is some evidence that babies who were induced prematurely due to pre-eclampsia or high blood pressure may cry more, as may pre-term babies who had breathing difficulties.[7]

Perhaps stress in pregnancy can lead to excessive crying in the early months.

Sensitive Children – Born, Not Made?

Anecdotal evidence from chiropractors who treat children with ADHD (Attention Deficit Hyperactivity Disorder) notes that many of them begin their lives with colic, while occupational therapists have also

DID YOU KNOW?
– Fussy babies are born, not made.
One experiment investigated newborn behaviour to see if it was possible to predict who would be a colicky baby. They asked nursery nurses to rate babies' cries at birth, but in fact they didn't find this related to later fussiness.[8] However, the babies whom these nurses had rated as more active and more attentive at birth were more likely to be classified as irritable by their parents at one month of age. Another piece of research found that weak foetal movements at 37 weeks' pregnancy were a good prediction of babies who cried at one, six and twelve weeks, and again concluded that some babies are born with temperaments that predispose them to cry.[9]

observed that children with poor sensory modulation abilities often have a history of colic.[10] But this sort of evidence is not conclusive, because if you have a child with ADHD or other problem, it is tempting to look at their infancy in a negative light and in order to be conclusive, research would need to compare these children with a control group of 'normal' children to see if there was significantly more colic in either group. Perhaps that research will be done soon.

The Sensitive Baby

Dr T Berry Brazelton was one of the first paediatricians to notice that some babies are hypersensitive, seemingly unable to cope with too much stimulation. He noticed that many of these had been through a stressful pregnancy.[11] Not all sensitive babies have typical colic patterns, in that some of these might fuss for many more than three months, without the peak at six weeks typical of other colicky babies.[12]

However, Dr Brazelton did feel that there was some sort of inevitability to it, and as it seemed to be a stage most babies go through, he reckoned there must be a purpose to it. His suggestion is that fussing is about organizing:

An immature nervous system can take in and utilize stimuli throughout the day, but there is always a little bit of overload. As the day proceeds, the increasingly overloaded nervous system begins to cycle in shorter and shorter sleep and feeding periods. Finally it blows off steam in the form of an active, fussy period.[13]

He suggests that the best approach with a sensitive baby is to react calmly and use one calming strategy at a time. Don't overload him by doing everything at once.

As you can see, perhaps it depends on why your baby has colic! If your baby is colicky because he is over-sensitive, it would be harder to stop the crying once it starts.

How to Survive a Sensitive or Colicky Baby

Sensitive babies may just need a very quiet and calm environment. Some of them may want to be held in close contact to their mums for seemingly hours on end, perhaps because it returns them to a calmer time, pre-birth. Denying such a baby's need for contact won't make the need go away. As we have seen, the baby whose cries are answered now, will later be the child confident enough to show his independence and curiosity.

> **DID YOU KNOW?**
> **– Colicky babies are harder to soothe.**
> One study found that sucrose water effectively calms crying newborns for at least four minutes, but this effect begins to wear off by the time the babies are six weeks old.[14] Interestingly, though, it was less effective for babies with colic, suggesting that some colicky babies are less able to stop crying once started.[15] However, another small but double-blind study did find sucrose effective as a treatment for infant colic (2 ml of 12 per cent sucrose given when crying).[16]

Even though, generally speaking, babies who are carried more, cry less,[17] studies of colicky babies have not found that increased carrying stops the crying, although it can help some babies.[18,19] So, while carrying and cuddling won't necessarily stop the crying, at least you are letting your baby know you are there. Remember that your baby won't mind who is doing the carrying and cuddling, so share the burden. A colicky baby is a nightmare – make sure you are not alone.

I would advise any parent to beg, borrow or steal one of those 'little automatic swings'. We have found them indispensable with both our babies. Neither baby has been really colicky, but Elizabeth did tend to cry for a couple of hours each afternoon. With her I found that taking her outside/to toddler groups, etc. worked, and came to the conclusion that some babies start to experience boredom very early on (from 2-3 weeks). She definitely seemed to want to 'look at a different ceiling/play gym' on many occasions.

– Hayley, mother of Elizabeth and Edward

~ Times Change ~ Answer – 1886 ~

Marion Harland, Common sense in the nursery, *in Christina Hardyment,* Dream Babies: Child-care From Locke to Spock *(Jonathan Cape, 1983)*

16

Treatments for Colic

~ Times change – does the advice stay the same? ~

Paternal neglect is one of the most abundant sources of domestic sorrow. The father toils early and late and finds no time to fulfil duties to his children.

Conventional Medicines

There are lots of drugs out there being sold for colic; how do you know which ones are effective and which ones are safe?

One of the biggest problems is that different babies probably have different reasons for being colicky, and most of the drugs sold over the counter assume that your baby has indigestion. Sedatives used to be widely sold, too, which would of course stop your baby crying, but would not cure the colic and were probably not particularly safe to use long term.

In a systematic review of all treatments for infantile colic,[1] only one drug was found to be effective, and that was Dicyclomine (Dicycloverine), which unfortunately has serious side-effects and is not recommended for babies under six months. The only drug without serious side-effects, Simethicone (Infacol) was not found to be effective. Simethicone claims to work by dispersing and preventing the formation of gas pockets in the intestinal tract, but there is no evidence that colicky infants have increased gas production,[2] and anyway even in infants with 'gas-related symptoms', there was no statistical significant improvement in a randomized double-blind study.[3] Lactase enzymes such as found in Colief drops were also found to have no effect.[4]

Complementary Therapies

While there are lots of treatments to try, most of them have not been subjected to rigorous scientific study – but then, as we have just seen, many of the drugs for sale have not really been established to be effective. If your baby is colicky, your need is probably to try everything possible, and the beauty of complementary therapies is that they are unlikely to have side-effects.

If you have never tried complementary medicine before, it may seem hard to choose which type of practitioner to visit. Some are trained in more than one type of therapy, and will offer whichever seems appropriate. Word of mouth recommendations are useful. Some therapists themselves may suggest that another form of complementary medicine is more appropriate for you or your baby.

Find out beforehand how much treatment will cost. Although it may seem expensive, remember your visit will probably last more than an hour. Some may lower their fees in cases of hardship. It is also worth asking your GP if he or she can refer you. Many GPs do now work alongside complementary practitioners, particularly in London and in fund-holding practices. Some private medical insurance will cover some or all of the costs of treatment by homoeopaths or osteopaths.

Most practitioners describe their treatments as 'complementary, not alternative'. They say there is no conflict between their therapies and the help your GP offers.

The main difference with complementary medicine is that it is 'holistic'. This means that practitioners will treat your baby as a whole person rather than focusing on her symptoms.

On your first consultation, they will take a detailed case history. Treatment will depend not only on the current problem, but also on any other illnesses your baby has had. The therapist will also want to encourage your baby's body to heal itself.

CRANIAL OSTEOPATHY

Osteopathy was the first complementary medicine to be recognized by the British Medical Association, and now has statutory recognition. It has been around since 1870, and is common in the UK and US. Cranial osteopathy developed as an offshoot in the 1930s.

Cranial osteopaths look for disturbance in the bones of the skull, and remedy these with gentle massage. The theory behind this treatment being used for babies is that, during labour the baby's skull is compressed, distorting and overlapping the skull bones. This is as it should be, and normally the moulding is reduced in the first few days after birth by crying (which raises intracranial pressure) and by suckling, which also moves the face bones.

If the moulding is extreme, though, through a very slow or difficult birth or perhaps by an assisted delivery (forceps or vacuum extraction) then the baby cannot undo the compression unaided, and the retained compression makes the baby more irritable; perhaps to the extent of giving the baby a headache. She cries more and prefers being picked up, as this decreases pressure on the head.

A quick birth can also affect the baby, as the head is not given time to adapt to the moulding pressures, so compression is too sudden. Caesarean babies apparently need the stimulation of temporal bones that vaginal delivery gives, and can also need treatment.

It is also suggested by cranial osteopaths that the nerve to the tongue can be affected so suckling is less effective, and the baby tires before she has had enough milk, so feeding is frequent and erratic.

Treatments are private, and a baby usually needs somewhere between two and six treatments, depending on the severity of the problem.

DID YOU KNOW?
– Fiddling with bones – perhaps it does work?

One study compared treating colicky babies using either Dimethicone or by having a chiropractor manipulate spine and pelvis. The study found that the babies did significantly better with manipulation than with Dimethicone, although the crying was also reduced with the drug. The researchers concluded that even though not all cases of colic are muscular-skeletal in origin, those that are may certainly benefit from treatment.[6]

A follow-up study,[7] however, comparing spinal manipulation only to no treatment at all, found no significant difference, although this study had some flaws, mostly in that the chiropractor examined and treated the babies on their own, took no case history, and only treated the babies twice, none of which would happen in a real situation. However, this study does tell us that there is more research work needed.

Cranial osteopathy is popular with many parents, and there's anecdotal evidence that it helps babies with colic. Only one study seems to have looked at this scientifically. Twenty-eight babies with colic in Gloucester and Cheltenham were referred for treatment, and were randomly assigned to have no treatment or to receive cranial osteopathy once a week for four weeks. The treated babies were found to cry less and to sleep better than the babies who were not treated.[5]

HOMOEOPATHY – 'LIKE CURES LIKE'

Have you heard of it? Arnica, a remedy for bruising, which is often recommended for labour, and for toddlers' knocks and bumps, is an over-the-counter homoeopathic remedy.

Homoeopathy has been with us since 1810. Many doctors in France and Germany practise it, but only a few hundred of UK GPs are qualified homoeopaths. The practitioner will take a detailed medical history, and work out your baby's emotional and constitutional type before prescribing specific remedies. These consist of a minute dose of a substance which would normally *cause* symptoms in a healthy person, the idea being to stimulate your baby's body's own healing power. Because the remedies are so diluted, there should be no side-effects.

For Colic
- **Chamomilla – when your baby is crotchety or irritable, and especially if she requires movement to sleep**
- **Pulsatilla – to calm your baby when she seems to need to be with you to sleep but cries if you move away**
- **Colocynthis – for when pressure on the tummy seems to help**
- **Magnesium phosphorica – when warmth is better than pressure.[8]**

ACUPUNCTURE/ACUPRESSURE – 'EAST MEETS WEST'

Have you heard of it? – The TENS machine is based on acupuncture, the idea being that it gives pain relief in labour by applying a current to acupuncture points. Seasickness bands may help relieve morning sickness or travel sickness by acupressure.

Acupuncture has been a fundamental part of Chinese medicine for at least 2,000 years. It starts with a Traditional Chinese Medicine diagnosis. With an adult, the therapist would use (disposable) needles at specific acupuncture points, but when treating babies the therapist will use pressure rather than needles. Some GPs also have a qualification in medical acupuncture.

HERBAL MEDICINE – 'AS OLD AS MANKIND ITSELF'

Have you heard of it? Raspberry leaf tea is a common herbal preparation used in late pregnancy to prepare for labour.

Outside the industrialized nations, 80 per cent of the world's population rely on herbs for health, drawing on the established healing properties of certain plants. Many modern drug companies, in fact, simply make use of these discoveries to create more potent remedies. Some herbalists prepare tinctures, herbal teas, ointments and creams themselves.

For Colic
- **Chaomomite – calming**
- **Peppermint – eases intestinal spasms**
- **Dill – soothes gas; used as gripe water**
- **Fennel – facilitates digestion**

Herbal medicine has had some rigorous testing; one study found that herbal tea (containing extracts of chamomile, vervain, liquorice, fennel and balm mint in a sucrose solution) was more effective than sucrose alone.[9]

My third baby cried almost constantly, when not feeding or asleep, for the first 12 weeks. I found that if he sucked on my little finger that would sooth him (he wouldn't take a dummy), so I used to carry him in a sling a lot with my finger in his mouth — not ideal when you have two other children under five, but better than having him cry all the time. I also used to breastfeed him a lot and he slept in our bed (as did my first two). Then one day he just stopped and has been a very happy baby ever since.

— Angela, mother of Alice, Mattie and Billy

~ Times Change ~ Answer – 1842 ~

Rev John C Abbott, The Mothers Magazine, *in Christina Hardyment,*
Dream Babies: Child-care From Locke to Spock *(Jonathan Cape, 1983)*

Sleeping

17

How Sleep Works for You

~ Times change – does the advice stay the same? ~
We went through fire and water almost in trying to procure for him a natural sleep. We swung him in blankets, wheeled him in little carts, walked the room with him by the hour, etc., but he always looked wide awake as if he did not need sleep.

We spend at least a third of our life asleep, and your baby may spend two-thirds of his early life asleep, yet why or how we sleep is something we rarely think about – except, of course, when we're sleep-deprived!

'Broken nights' is probably one of your biggest fears when you're expecting a baby. It's such an emotive phrase – why is your night 'broken'? You might as well face it now: it is completely inevitable that your baby will wake during the night – but as you will see, the impact this has on you depends on several things, including where you are in your sleep cycle, and how you decide to respond to your baby's needs during the night.

Adult Sleep

The first step towards getting a good night's sleep is to understand why you need to sleep, how your sleep works, and how your baby's sleep fits in with this.

We adults need an average of eight hours sleep per night. However, no one sleeps for eight hours at a stretch; our sleep is cyclical, with each cycle lasting about 90 to 100 minutes; therefore, in eight hours you will have five cycles or 'stages'.

Each cycle starts with non-rapid-eye-movement (NREM) sleep, which comprises firstly two phases of light sleep and then two phases of deep sleep. After that, you move briefly back into light sleep before descending into a different type of sleep, called rapid-eye-movement (REM) sleep. You wake up briefly from this, and then the whole cycle repeats.

THE FIVE STAGES OF ADULT SLEEP

NREM, *Light Sleep – Stage One*
This is the initial phase of sleep. Your muscles start to relax; if you are sitting up, your head slumps forward, your mouth drops open – you're 'nodding off'. It's easy for you to wake from this stage; you might not even realize you've been asleep. This is why driving when you are sleepy is particularly dangerous; many sleep-deprived people have nodded off into Stage-one sleep and crashed without ever realizing they were asleep.

> **WHAT IS SLEEP FOR?**
> We now believe that REM sleep is about allowing our brains to process information – a bit like a night-time filing and storage system, while deep, NREM sleep allows the body to rest and physically repair itself. Pituitary growth hormones, which are responsible for growth and repair, peak during NREM.[1]

 116 Step Three: Sleeping

Stage one sleep lasts only a few minutes.

NREM, Light Sleep – Stage Two – 'Spindle' Sleep

You're more relaxed during Stage Two; you're less easily woken, and you appear to be sound asleep. You're not yet dreaming. This phase is called 'spindle sleep' because when scientists recorded the brain-waves of people at this point in light sleep, they reckoned that the trace looked like a spindle moving along a loom.

Adults spend 45-50 per cent of the night in light, spindle sleep.

NREM, Deep Sleep – Stage Three – Slow-wave Sleep

About 10 or 15 minutes after you fall asleep, deep sleep begins with Stage Three; your brain waves are now slow and rolling.

NREM Deep Sleep – Stage Four – Slow-wave Sleep

Stage Four is the deepest form of sleep, with even slower brain waves. You are deeply relaxed and it's very hard to wake you up. The first time in the night that you enter Stage Four sleep, you will probably be in it for at least half an hour.

You spend about 25 per cent of your night in slow-wave deep sleep (Stages Three and Four).

REM Sleep

After being asleep for about an hour, having experienced light sleep, deep sleep and moving very briefly into light sleep again, your brain waves go mad, and it looks as if you have woken up, but in fact you are in REM sleep.

During REM sleep, your eyes move rapidly, hence the name – Rapid Eye Movement sleep. Your breathing sounds irregular, you use up energy. Your body is motionless, for good reason – you are now experiencing your most vivid dreams, and if you were able to move you might well start enacting them! If someone wakes you up now, you would probably say you were dreaming and would be able to remember the dream. It is easier to wake you up at this stage of sleep than from deep sleep.

All adults have up to two hours of REM sleep per night.

Research suggests that the most important part of our night's rest is REM sleep, as this lets your brain 'process and file' everything that you have learned and experienced that day. Long-term REM deprivation makes people depressed and disorganized.

Being woken from NREM sleep makes us tired but able to cope the following day. However, if our REM sleep is disturbed, we find the next day much harder. When someone is deprived of sleep for several nights, the percentage of REM sleep increases dramatically during the catch-up nights.[3]

At the end of each complete cycle, you actually wake up, make a brief check of your surroundings and, if everything is normal, you fall asleep again. This is why you often sleep badly when you are in a strange place; at the end of each sleep cycle, instead of going back down towards deep sleep again, you awake fully, disturbed by being in an unfamiliar place, so you then need to get sleepy again.

DID YOU KNOW?
– Sleeping makes you brainy!
In one experiment, men were taught Morse code shortly before they went to bed, and researchers noticed that they then had longer and more frequent REM episodes. Another experiment found that for English-speaking students learning French, those who were best at learning the new language had the biggest increases in REM sleep. However, REM sleep does need to happen fairly soon after learning for any new skills to be remembered.[2]

REM sleep does not happen equally throughout the night, though. As the night progresses, your REM sleep becomes longer and your slow-wave sleep becomes shorter, so that in a typical night you have slow-wave, physically refreshing sleep early in the night, and REM sleep in the early morning. So if you get enough sleep and can wake naturally in the morning, you will be waking from the end of your last phase of REM sleep, and should feel both physically and mentally refreshed.

This 90-minute sleep cycle is not unique to our nights; we have a basic rest-activity cycle (BRAC) during the day, where we move from being alert and efficient through to not concentrating and being spaced out, and guess what? These are about 90 minutes long. Not being able to concentrate for long periods is natural; we have periods where we lose focus, stop attending and become reflective, and these 'tuning out' times may be restorative, just like REM sleep.

What Happens to Your Sleep When You Have a Baby?

If your sleep is disrupted mid-cycle, your metabolic rate rises, so that you use up more energy even if you end up with roughly the same amount of sleep. So if you are getting out of bed every few hours to look after a baby, even if you still end up with eight hours sleep in total, you will be physically more tired.

It's a good idea to take the odd catnap during the day. Even if you don't sleep, the physical rest will help.

Becoming a parent involves learning many new skills, so it would be better if new mothers and fathers did not miss out on their REM sleep, given that REM is important for consolidating learning experiences and remembering things. One researcher also suggested that our self-confidence, our ability to remain optimistic and to adapt emotionally to our physical and social environment is also affected by REM sleep[4] – important for new parents who may be coping on their own without support from an extended family.

Getting out of bed to look after a baby in the night will be tiring, and will affect you physically and mentally. But we would not have lasted long as a species if new mothers were so chronically sleep-deprived they failed to avoid the sabre-toothed tiger, or if fathers could not concentrate on catching that night's dinner. Nature has allowed for the fact that we have to look after babies *and* function during the day, and we will see more of how this is meant to work in the next few chapters.

Interestingly, men's testosterone levels, which get depleted during the day, are topped up during sleep, reaching a peak around dawn. So if fathers have to spend the early hours of the day awake and looking after babies, it will certainly affect their sex drives; however, new mothers might wonder whether this is a good or a bad thing!

My baby suffered very badly from colic and I would spend hours pacing the house rocking him in my arms. To make the whole process more bearable I placed a glass of wine on the table and every time I completed a circuit I would have a sip!

– *Zoya, mother to Charlie*

~ Times Change ~ Answer – 1833 ~

From G L Prentiss, The Life and letters of Elizabeth Prentiss – *in Paul Martin*, Counting Sheep *(HarperCollins, 2001)*

18

How Sleep Works for Your Baby

~ Times change – does the advice stay the same? ~

Left to his own devices, a baby will drift easily in and out of sleep as his body requires it – but scarcely any child in the West is left to his own devices.

Newborn babies can sleep for 16 out of 24 hours; so why do parents have such difficulty coping? Because it's not the *amount* of time she spends asleep that causes the problem, but her sleep cycle, which is fundamentally different to yours.

Your Baby's Sleep – How It Develops

WHILE YOU ARE PREGNANT

Before she was born, your baby spent 60 to 80 per cent of her time in rapid-eye-movement (REM) sleep. We don't know why this is, but one suggestion is that perhaps REM sleep gives her visual images to help her brain develop properly despite the lack of visual stimulation.[1] Foetuses and very young babies do not have non-NREM 1-4 and REM sleep as we do. Instead, they have essentially just two types of sleep:

1 Active or REM sleep
2 Quiet, which develops into NREM sleep.

THE FIRST FEW WEEKS

Your baby will have so many new experiences after she is born, she needs lots of REM sleep to help process them, but she also needs NREM sleep time to conserve physical energy so she can grow. It's been estimated that if a child continued to grow at the same rate throughout her childhood as she does in these early months, she would be the height of Nelson's column by the time she left home!

After she is born, she will, therefore, sleep a lot. It is not easy to work out exactly how much sleep a baby needs, as throughout history the amount cited has been mostly based on childcare fashions, and not from any real understanding of a baby's physiology. During the last century, for instance, when babies were expected to spend most of their life asleep in a pram at the bottom of the garden, it was not uncommon to read that babies needed as much as 24 hours of sleep a day (yes, you did read that correctly!).[2]

Also, as James McKenna, sleep researcher and anthropologist[3] points out, much of what we know about babies' sleep physiology has been deduced from non-breastfeeding, solitary sleeping babies – and neither of these conditions are biologically or socially normal, as you will see later on (pages 158–64).

What we currently think is that newborn babies need on average 12 to 16 hours of sleep in 24, which sounds great – but as this happens in 60-minute cycles, and as 50 per cent of her sleep is REM and the other 50 per cent is light NREM sleep, it means that she will wake frequently, potentially rousing every hour. As your natural cycle is 90 minutes long, you can see that your baby starts life in a completely different rhythm.

Some young babies can stay asleep during light sleep and at the end of their 60-minute cycle, but many will drift in and out of sleep fairly ineffectively, depending on their ability to soothe themselves.

Interestingly, babies who are born pre-term actually have less REM sleep, but by the time they reach their due date, it rapidly increases. Presumably pre-term babies need to spend more time in NREM sleep to help them grow.

AT SIX WEEKS

During her first six weeks, your baby's circadian rhythm, which governs heart rate, temperature and activity level, matures so that she begins to develop a pattern that helps her to be asleep or awake effectively, rather than just drifting between these states. Somewhere between one

DID YOU KNOW?
– Babies in the womb know about night and day!

Contrary to popular belief, babies do have diurnal (night and day) rhythms. Before they are born, their mother's hormones tell them when it is day or night.[4] After birth, when they are not subject to these, they lose this for a bit and need a few weeks to set up their own circadian rhythms, but they do tend to sleep slightly more at night; even babies a few weeks old do most of their sleeping between midnight and 4 a.m., and most of their crying and fussing between 4 p.m. and 8 p.m., with an additional peak between 8 a.m. and noon, though this extra fussy period tends to disappear by the fourth week. There is also a progressive drop in both the average feeding and fussing/crying times by week eight, reflecting increased settled and awake periods.[5]

and three months of age you may see her pattern developing, so that she should sleep less frequently, but for longer periods. It can help to keep a note of her sleeping patterns to give you an idea of how they're developing.

Whether your baby is sleeping with you or alone will also affect her arousal patterns, as we will see in the next section.

AT FOUR MONTHS

Although babies over four months probably need the same amount of sleep as they did when they were newborn, what happens with many babies is that these sleep episodes start to join up, so that they might sleep for a few hours at a stretch during the night, and have longer periods awake during the day.

DID YOU KNOW?
– Birth affects sleep.
Interestingly, one study found a difference between baby's diurnal patterns depending on whether they had been born vaginally or by c-section. Babies born by c-section seemed to lack a diurnal sleep rhythm, regardless of whether the Caesarean was emergency or elective, suggesting that it was the surgical intervention which interfered with the baby's natural diurnal pattern.[6]

By three or four months you may find that your baby is awake during the late afternoon and early evening, tending to sleep twice as much at night as during the day. She will also be alert for longer periods; the longest awake-time for the average four-month-old increases to about eight hours.

In addition, her sleep cycle will begin to resemble yours, being capable of having more defined Stage three and four (deep) sleep, though the whole cycle will still be shorter, and there will still be more REM episodes. By this age, too, most of the REM sleep will be at night, and her daytime sleep will tend to be NREM. Not all babies, of course, adapt to this pattern.[7]

How Sleep Works for Your Baby 125 ♡

AT SIX MONTHS

Sometime around six months of age, babies' REM sleep drops from the initial 50 per cent to resemble the adult levels of around 25 per cent. The sleep cycle also increases from the initial 60 minutes to the adult 90 minutes. So by now, your baby's sleep patterns should resemble yours.

When Might My Baby Sleep Through the Night?

It is worth pointing out that the official definition of a baby 'sleeping through the night' used in sleep research is that the baby should sleep from midnight to 5 a.m., not for 12 or 14 hours at a stretch. Although researchers have found that 85 per cent of babies can sleep through by six months, and you may hear this quoted, do bear in mind that this means five hours of sleep, not eight or even twelve!

What we would hope is that by six months (four months if you're lucky), your baby will sleep for a significant block of time at night, with a couple of daytime naps. By one year old, your baby will need about two daytime naps and a long period of sleep at night; by two years, your baby will probably only have one daytime nap, but this will still be a reasonably long one – anywhere between one and three hours. Even so, it is not at all unusual for babies to wake during their night time sleeps; a national survey of English mothers found that a quarter of one-year-olds were still waking during the night at least five nights a week.[8]

It is useful to remember that *none* of us sleeps through the night – we all wake up every 90 minutes, and your baby will wake every 60 minutes until she is a few months old. Most of us, though, are able to go back to sleep unaided; so the question is not 'when will my baby sleep through the night?', but 'when will she stop needing my help to get back to sleep?'

Some young babies are capable of 'self-soothing' early on, but many babies need help for quite some time.

The other issue, of course, is that young babies do need to be fed during the night and day, so until she no longer needs to be fed at night, she will wake. Of course, it's not always easy to work out when this time arrives, as night-waking can become more about comfort and needing you to help her get back to sleep than actually about hunger. We will look at all these issues in the next few chapters.

For the first couple of months Luke pretty much ate and slept when he wanted. By the time he was six months old his milk feeds and solid meals were at roughly the same time each day, but he still slept whenever he wanted or as our schedule allowed. His sleeps do vary in length according to what we've been doing and how tired he is, but at about four months he was sleeping for about 10 hours a night, and soon after was sleeping for 12 hours (unless he was teething!).

Luke is pretty easy-going, so he may have fitted into a stricter routine if I had wanted him to, but I felt it was more important for him to be flexible. Also, as our activities are at different times every day, so I couldn't have coped with a rigid routine.

Julie – mother of Luke

~ Times Change ~ Answer – 1999 ~
From Deborah Jackson, Three in a Bed *(Bloomsbury, 1999)*

19

Can You Train Your Baby to Sleep Through the Night?

~ Times change – does the advice stay the same? ~

It is a serious question in my mind whether children should know their own parents at all. There are undoubtedly much more scientific ways of bringing up children.

We probably all like the idea of being able to teach our babies to sleep through the night. You've probably heard of 'controlled crying' – leaving babies to cry – and how this can get your baby to sleep longer. But does it really work? Before I answer that question, let's take a look at how the idea evolved.

Behaviourism, or Learning Theory

One of the earliest forms of learning to be studied by psychologists came to be called Classical Conditioning. You've probably vaguely heard of Pavlov's dogs. Pavlov was a Russian physiologist working in the 1920s, investigating dog's saliva (well, someone had to do it!). He noticed that the dogs in his laboratory started to salivate when they saw the bucket which normally contained their food; even before the food arrived. As dogs normally only salivate at the sight, smell or taste of food, Pavlov realized that the dogs were *associating* (making a connection between) the bucket with food, and went on to investigate whether they could learn to associate other objects with food. He started ringing bells at meal times, and within a few sessions, the dogs would salivate whenever they heard a bell.

This is Classical Conditioning, where food is an Unconditional Stimulus (works every time), salivation being an Unconditional Response (ditto); the bell becomes a Conditional Stimulus, and salivation at the sound of a bell is a Conditional Response (so the response has been *learned*).

Each time the dog gets fed after the bell rings is called *reinforcement*. If the bell rings and there is no food, there is no reinforcement, and over time the Conditional Response fades; a process known as *extinction*.

From this work, a whole branch of psychology developed called Behaviourism, which believed that all human learning was about conditioning. One of its leading proponents, John Watson, wrote books about childcare in the 1920s based on these principles, and did a few unpleasant experiments on children, including one on a little boy called Albert.

When Albert was 11 months old, Watson paired the loud noise made by a hammer with the appearance of a white rat, and indeed discovered that Albert developed a fear of white rats. Over time, this *generalized* to a fear of other similar objects such as rabbits, dogs and even cotton wool.

Behaviourism has gone out of fashion now, and its principles are only used today in treating addictions or phobias – and in trying to get children to sleep!

Behaviourism in Managing Baby's Sleep

The theory behind sleep-training of this kind is that when a baby is fed during the night, his waking becomes *associated* with getting attention from his parent, so that even when he no longer needs to feed at night, the waking has been *reinforced*. Once the need for food at night has passed, if the baby is still waking it is assumed that waking has become *associated* with a pleasant outcome – usually some form of social contact, though as you can see with Albert and his fear of cotton wool, it is not always obvious how associations develop.

Behaviourism and sleep-training are about working out what the waking has become associated with, and then either removing the reinforcing consequences of the waking or setting up new associations so that parents' presence is no longer needed.

The way to stop the waking can involve one of several techniques:

- **Extinction**
- **Fading**
- **Reinforcement**
- **Cueing**

Extinction

This is the most famous and perhaps most notorious form of behaviour modification; we know it as 'controlled crying', and it's about not

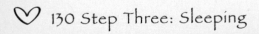

responding when your child cries out in the night, the idea being that the rewarding effect of your attention is removed.

Some therapists allow you to go and check that the child is 'all right', but you are not allowed to interact with them, as you will be reinforcing their behaviour again. Eventually, the theory goes, the baby will stop crying because the association is *extinguished*.

The advantage of this method is that the problem will be solved quickly – the baby will give up crying. The disadvantage is that it is hard on both parent and child, as it will involve several nights of crying for hours. Parents also have to be aware that if at any point they give in and pick the child up, they will have reinforced the behaviour again and be back to square one.

I would suggest that this is only appropriate for older children, where you can explain what you are doing, and only when you know the child is capable of getting himself to sleep.

Fading

The idea here is to change the baby's behaviour by *gradually* removing the stimulus which is *associated* with the behaviour.

Examples are:

For a baby who wakes in the night and needs to be mothered to sleep:

1 Going from holding, rocking or feeding the baby to sleep, through just sitting next to the baby or perhaps stroking him, then sitting next to him, then moving to the door, to standing outside the door, and so on.

Can You Train Your Baby to Sleep Through 131

For a child who will not go to bed at a reasonable time:

2 Starting bedtime routines later in evening when the baby is more likely to settle, and then gradually moving bedtime forward.

The advantages of fading as a technique is that it does not involve leaving a baby to cry on his own. The disadvantage is that it can take a long time.

I would suggest this as a good strategy for parents who have an older baby with sleep problems, when you can see where you are going wrong, and just want to change this without distressing your baby.

Reinforcement

This is a more positive type of behaviour modification – to go back to dogs for a minute, it's like giving a dog a biscuit for good behaviour, for instance. If we apply this to babies, then we are trying to reinforce good behaviour by external rewards.

Reinforcement does work really well with children; but usually only those of a certain age. They need to be fluent speakers, for a start, as you need to explain what you are doing. In the context of sleep, you could offer a reward to your toddler for staying in his own bed all night, or for not waking you up and so on, but it is hard to see how this would be effective for babies.

I would suggest using this with much older children, who are already familiar with star charts and the like.

Cueing

This is also a positive form of behaviour modification, involving strengthening or altering the *cues* which are associated with going to sleep. When sleeping difficulties occur, the parents usually provide a *cue* which helps the infant fall asleep, such as a key word, a special place and so on. *Cueing* is what we use when we try to establish a bedtime routine, as you will see in the next chapter.

This is one of the most effective techniques to use with young babies, and as it involves working with your baby's natural sleep cycles, there is no crying.

Does Behaviourism Really Work?

Behaviourism went out of fashion in most areas of child development – except sleep! – as we now know that human beings are far more complicated than dogs, for instance. The behaviourists of the 1920s, who developed these ideas, did not believe that human beings had any sort of innate, internal emotional life. They believed that we were born 'blank slates' and that everything we became later in life was a result of conditioning.

We now know that babies are indeed born with a complex

DID YOU KNOW?
– Babies who have problematic births are more likely to have sleeping difficulties later. Children who have sleep problems have often had problems in the womb, at labour and at birth. Mild asphyxia at birth is associated with a failure to sleep through the night at three months, and children who are still having sleep problems at five years of age are more likely to have been born to women admitted to hospital during pregnancy or those who had an assisted delivery (forceps or vacuum extraction).[1]

Can You Train Your Baby to Sleep Through 133

intelligence, that they are capable of many things without being taught, and that both babies and adults have emotional needs and an emotional intelligence which simple learning theory cannot explain.

The core assumption in learning theory and sleep-training is that babies are perfectly capable of sleeping on their own, and that the difficulties they have are maintained (if not caused by) the actions of the parents. It also assumes that crying is a negative behaviour which should be extinguished, nothing more.

However, it is worth pointing out that at a young age, crying is a baby's only means of communication. If we take account of the world from the baby's point of view – if we consider the meaning of our actions from his perspective – not responding to his cries is, in effect, ignoring what he is trying to say. It has been argued that leaving a baby to cry:

- **takes away his desire to communicate**
- **makes him lose trust in you**
- **could damage your baby's emerging self-esteem.**

It has also been argued that young babies are not ready to sleep through the night (not alone, anyway).

Most people who favour extinction as a method claim it does work – that the baby will eventually stop crying out in the night. But we don't really know what the long-term effect of this short-term gain is likely to be.

There has been some research to evaluate the effectiveness of the behavioural management approach to sleep-training, and on the whole, sleep-training techniques do not bear up under research.

In studies comparing a control group (where no training takes place) to an intervention group (having some form of behaviour training), there has not always been a significant difference between the two. Other studies, without a control group, have reported a success rate of about 50 per cent, but in fact one would expect about half of the children in any sample to improve over time, without intervention.[2]

The most recent systematic review (where researchers review all other research that has been done in the field) noticed that both extinction and positive bedtime routines seem to be effective compared to drugging children, for instance, but that on the whole the methodology of most studies is poor, and many parents dislike the interventions, which of course would affect how strictly they went along with the routine. The overall conclusion from this systematic review, which is common sense really, is that 'choice of treatment needs to be based on the families' preferences and circumstances.'[3]

The studies where behavioural management does seem to work are those where there is a skilled therapist involved, helping parents on an individual basis.[4] This makes intuitive sense: if you are in the middle of a problem, and emotionally involved, it is not always easy to assess the best way forward.

Even if you do believe that your baby is waking up due to a conditional response, reinforced by your behaviour, turning this around is not easy to do on your own. The behavioural management techniques may look as if they should work, but they have not always been shown to be effective, and it does take skill to identify the causes of your child's sleeping difficulties and to identify the appropriate remedy. You will also need support to keep going. Sleep clinics, which your health visitor can refer you to, are a good place to get this sort of practical help and support.

In addition, research seems to suggest that different techniques work better at different stages, so that's worth thinking about when choosing an appropriate strategy for your baby.

Our first child used to wake every two hours during the night, and was still doing so when he was 18 months old. As it turned out, we were reinforcing his waking behaviour, but being inexperienced parents and fuddled from lack of sleep, we didn't see this until we attended a sleep clinic, filled in a sleep diary for two weeks, and had the health visitor point out exactly what our reinforcing behaviours were.

Within three days of this Sword of Damocles experience, our baby was sleeping through the night, having never slept more than two hours before, and we never needed to leave him to cry, either – we just had to stop the reinforcing behaviour. But if we had left him to cry, even at 18 months, it would have been cruel because he had no resources of his own to get to sleep – we had trained him to fall asleep with a conditional response!

– *Caroline, mother to Alasdair, Chris and Josie – and author of this book!*

~ Times Change ~ Answer – 1928 ~

From J B Watson, Psychological Care of Infant and Child –
father of behaviourism!

20

Helping Your Baby Fall Asleep

~ Times change – does the advice stay the same? ~

*A child should never be compelled to endure caresses, never
overwhelmed with kisses, which ordinarily torment him and are
often the cause of sexual hyperæsthesia. The child's demonstrations
of affection should be reciprocated when they are sincere, but one's
own demonstrations should be reserved for special occasions.*

Most parents find that there are two main sleep issues for babies,
and you will probably grapple with one or both at various times in
your child's life! These are:

1 falling asleep
2 staying asleep.

In this chapter, we look at how to encourage your baby to fall asleep
on her own, and in the following chapter we'll consider how to help
her stay asleep for longer periods.

Research into sleep training consistently shows that the most effective strategy early on is to find a way of establishing the difference between night and day for your baby,[1] and this involves two things:

- **When you feed your baby at night, keep the lights dim, talk quietly – avoid too much interaction – basically communicate that this is sleep time. Don't change her nappy unless she is dirty.**
- **Establish a bedtime routine that will involve *cues* to let her know it is time to sleep.**

It really doesn't matter what you do or when you do it, as long as you try to do the same thing every day. Your aim is to get your baby to associate certain rituals with falling asleep. Having said that, some rituals will be more effective than others, and again it is useful to look at adult sleep and to understand what helps us to slip into the land of nod.

How to Fall Asleep

We grown-ups do not lie down in bed and instantly fall asleep, unless we're severely sleep-deprived. The amount of time it takes you to fall asleep is called your 'sleep latency'.

A drop in body temperature is one of the most important 'triggers' for sleep. Normally your core body temperature drops just before you nod off, so your body temperature has a big effect on your sleep latency. That's why it's hard to get to sleep if you're too hot.

You have probably already discovered for yourself that you can make this work for you, by taking a hot bath an hour or two before you want to sleep. The hot bath raises your temperature briefly, so that when you get out and your temperature starts to drop, you feel sleepy.

- **A nice warm bath as part of your baby's bedtime ritual
  will help her sleep, as long as she enjoys being bathed.
  See 'Making Baths Less Scary' (page 80) for tips on helping
  her enjoy her bath.**

As you probably know from being outside on a cold day, to conserve
your core body temperature your body stops circulating blood to your
extremities, so your hands and feet get cold. So you can use reverse
physiology. In order to cool your core body temperature and thus trig-
ger sleep, warm up your hands and feet!

Have you ever lain awake for hours because your feet were cold?
That's why wearing bed-socks or putting a hot water bottle at your
feet is so effective! It also means that artificially warming the centre
of your bed with a hot water bottle or electric blanket can disturb
your sleep. In addition, physical exercise or a large meal close to bedtime will raise your core body temperature and keep you awake.[2]

- **Make sure your baby's hands and feet are warm enough.
  You can put a hot water bottle at the foot of her cot before
  she goes to bed, but take it out before she gets in to avoid
  overheating.**

DEVELOPING A HAPPY BEDTIME ROUTINE

Your routine needs to involve winding down, so start with a bath,
then after a clean nappy and perhaps special bedtime clothes, give
her a milk feed and finally, tuck her up in her cot – remember not to
put her in an adult bed alone. Some parents like to give their baby a
massage after the bath; others may just have a nice cuddle. It does-
n't really matter what you choose to do; a bedtime routine is basically about keeping things predictable.

Over time, the bedtime ritual will in itself make her dozy, but before
she is used to this, you may have to time it carefully to coincide with

a sleepy period. This might mean starting preparations when she's fully awake so that she is ready for tucking in as a sleep phase approaches.

You can develop some key words, like 'nighty-night' to cue sleep; the idea being that eventually she will associate them with falling asleep. To get these to work effectively, use them when bedtime is going well, so they become associated with happily falling asleep, and not, for instance, with feeling agitated.

FALLING ASLEEP IN YOUR ARMS

Babies will often fall asleep while feeding, whether at the breast or bottle. Some mothers are quite happy for this to happen, and in the early days, when your baby is drifting between alert and asleep phases, it is hard to see that you could do any different. However, if your baby always falls asleep while feeding, it may be that in time she associates the two, and begins to feel the need to feed in order to fall asleep.

In addition, if you are intending to sleep apart from your baby, if she falls asleep in your arms or at your breast, when she wakes briefly at the end of a sleep cycle she will be startled awake by the fact that you are no longer there, just as would happen to you if you woke to find yourself somewhere different than when you dropped off. So while it is fine to 'mother' her to sleep sometimes, by feeding or rocking, it's also a good idea to aim to put your baby down for the night when she is dozing off, but before she is fully asleep, on most occasions.

NOISES OFF

What happens when you put her down, leave the room, and she starts to make a noise? Remember that she is learning to get herself to sleep, and as we saw when we talked about sleep latency, she will probably not fall asleep immediately. Some books suggest leaving your baby to cry, but most parents react against this, and luckily current research supports them, as you saw in the last chapter.

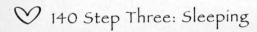

However, do listen to the type of cry your baby is making. Is it a moany, grumpy, tired cry that might mean she's trying to fall asleep? Some mothers go on picking their baby up every time they make the slightest noise, when sometimes it might be better to hang on. If the cry comes when you know she's tired, try leaving her for a couple of minutes, only picking her up if the cry changes or becomes more urgent. You could try instead giving her a little stroke or other quiet, gentle reassurance.

Obviously you must do what you feel comfortable doing, and if you think she sounds upset, fearful or anxious, then go back, comfort her, and if you can, settle her again to sleep. Parenting is about confidence – if you act undecided, or seem fearful about leaving her to fall asleep, she will believe you and think there really is something to worry about!

PEACE AND QUIET
One of the most common misconceptions about babies is that they need silence to get to sleep. Can you imagine how complete silence must sound to a baby who has spent nine months surrounded by the racket of her mother's womb? In time, yes, your baby will learn to sleep when it is quiet, but if you make this your goal now, you may be creating a rod for your own back. Do you want to be stuck indoors because your baby needs a daytime nap in utter silence? Isn't it better if she can sleep while you shop, visit friends and generally get on with your life?

The Importance of Daytime Naps

How your baby naps during the day will affect her ability to sleep at night. If she is having difficulty falling asleep at bedtime, then it's worth having a think about the quality and quantity of her daytime naps.

Too Late in the Afternoon?

Try to let her sleep no later than 3 p.m. if you want a bedtime around 6 or 7 p.m.

Too Long in the Day?

Is she sleeping for too long in the day? Or perhaps, not long enough! Ironically, if your baby does not get the sleep she needs during the day, she might be overtired by bedtime and too cranky to settle well.

A ROUGH GUIDE

4 months	Up to three daytime naps, total time probably maximum 4 hours
6 months	One morning nap for about 1 hour and one after lunch, maximum 2 hours
12 months	She may have dropped the morning nap, she may not, but she will definitely need an after-lunch nap of around 2 hours
2 years	After-lunch nap, 1 to 2 hours
3 years	After-lunch nap, about 1 hour
4 years	No naps

Use Her Natural Cycles

As we have learned, we all have basic rest/activity cycles (BRAC), so try to take advantage of your baby's own natural cycles of being alert or being at rest. Look out for signs of tiredness so you can act upon these before she gets crotchety, especially to make the most of a daytime nap. For a baby, these signs might include:

- avoiding eye-contact
- looking glazed, out of focus
- fussing
- rubbing her eyes
- yawning.

For an older child, these are some of the signs:

- a lull in movement or activity
- quieting down
- losing interest in other people or toys.

Two brilliant aids were firstly a lambskin rug which Samuel has slept on since he was about a month old. It has always been a great comfort to him – he adores it. The second was a sleeping bag. He would always end up kicking off the blankets, as he was quite fidgety in his cot, and of course this would wake him up when he got cold. After putting him in a 100-per cent cotton sleeping bag (at about 3 months), his wakings reduced to only feed times and we won ourselves some well-earned extra sleep! At 16 months he still sleeps in a sleeping bag and snoozes uninterrupted for usually 12 hours – 7 p.m. to 7 a.m. Hope these tips help someone else as obsessed with getting enough sleep as I am!

– *Andrea, mother to Samuel*

~ Times Change ~ Answer – 1910 ~
From Ellen Key, The Education of the Child *(Electronic Text Center, University of Virginia Library)*

21

Helping Your Baby Stay Asleep

~ Times change – does the advice stay the same? ~

*If you find that you actually prefer to have your child in your bed,
you should examine your feelings very carefully.*

'My baby slept through from six weeks …' is a variation on one of the most unhelpful statements you will hear. Immediately you feel inadequate, but remember – no six-week-old baby sleeps from 7 p.m. to 7 a.m., for instance, without stirring. Sometimes a baby will sleep for a long stretch a few nights running and their parents think they've cracked it, but unfortunately it rarely lasts. Whatever the truth, the only important fact is whether *you* feel happy with your baby's sleep patterns.

What Do We Know about Physiology?

As we have already seen, no one, including your baby, falls asleep and stays in the same level of sleep. We all wake briefly, several times

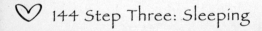

a night. When your baby wakes, he won't necessarily turn over and go straight back to sleep, unless he feels that it is safe to do so. If, however, you have become a necessary part of his sleeping routine, he will need you each time he wakes.

The Art of Getting a Baby to Sleep Through

1 Teach him to fall asleep by himself. We looked, in the previous chapter, at doing this with the first sleep of the night. We also saw there how important it was that your baby is able to fall asleep without being 'mothered' to sleep, if you want him to sleep happily on his own.

2 Help him to decide that it's OK to go back to sleep when he wakes up. If he is already capable of falling asleep unaided, then the next step is for him to decide to do this in the dead of night.

Making the Night Different from the Day

Remember that your baby is first and foremost a social creature, and he wants to please you, his parents, and to do whatever you and the society he lives in want him to do, as long as this does not conflict with his deeper and more basic needs, such as the need to feed, sleep and feel safe.

What you would like him to understand is that night-time is for sleep, daytime is for being awake. Even as a young baby he already has rudimentary diurnal cycles (night and day) as well as developing rhythms of arousal and sleep, so you are not going against his nature in encouraging him to sleep at night. However, he will be incapable of sleeping if:

- he is hungry or thirsty, and for the first three or four months he will need feeding during the night
- he is afraid. If he feels he has been abandoned, he will need your presence.

NIGHT-FEEDING

Given that he will need to feed at night as well as during the day in his first few months, you can use these night feeds as a way of teaching him that night-time is different. So, when you feed him at night:

- Keep the room as dark as possible. You might like to use a nightlight if he is not in bed with you so you can see what you're doing, but if he is in bed and you are breastfeeding, you may well find, with a couple of weeks' practice, that you can both do it in the dark with your eyes shut!
- Don't change his nappy at night (unless he is dirty). Babies don't mind being wet.
- Keep everything low-key. Don't start socializing; whisper or murmur if you need to speak to him. Bore him back to sleep if need be!

Research has suggested that this intervention – that is, emphasizing day and night differences and minimizing interactions at night – is effective. In one study of over 600 babies, it led to a 10 per cent increase in the number of babies at 12 weeks of age who slept for 5 or more hours at night (the definition, if you remember, of 'sleeping through the night'!)[1]

REASSURANCE

If your baby is sleeping with you, then he is unlikely to need reassurance during the night – he knows he is safe. If he is sleeping on his own, and you know that he is capable of falling asleep on his own without being fed, rocked or whatever, because he can already do this at bedtime, then when he wakes at night and can't fall asleep again, he probably just needs reassurance that you are still there somewhere, and that his cot is still a safe place to be.

- **If your baby wakes more often than you think he needs to, have a think about what you are doing when he wakes up. Does it reinforce his waking – is it worth him waking for? Lots of singing, dancing and cuddling is worth waking for, but a brief, unexciting reassurance is not.**
- **If your baby is older and is capable of going for longer stretches between feeds, yet you always feed him when he wakes, again this may be making it more worth his while to wake up than to turn over and go back to sleep. You could try a bottle of water, or just a reassurance instead. It can also be helpful if someone else can go to him until he gets used to not being fed.**

It is always easier and safer for him to sleep in your room in the first months; once he no longer needs a night feed he may sleep better in his room on his own.

SHOULD I LEAVE HIM TO CRY IT OUT?
We've looked at the principles and practice of behavioural adaptation training earlier, and have seen that the idea behind leaving a baby to cry is that he already knows how to fall asleep on his own, he is just choosing not to, and leaving him to cry is giving him the message that it is easier to choose to fall asleep because you are not going to make it worthwhile him being awake.

If your baby is not yet capable of falling asleep on his own, then this is not going to work, and although eventually he will stop crying through sheer exhaustion, there is no positive lesson to be learned. Before you try any of these techniques, you need to be sure that your baby can fall asleep on his own quite happily.

If Your Baby Starts to Wake More Frequently at Night

Is something affecting him right now? Any major changes such as moving house or his mum starting back at work may affect his sleep. If he is ill or teething, you can expect unsettled nights. Remember, no one's child sleeps through every night, so be calm, persevere, and he will sleep through again.

Some of the reasons your baby might have problems sleeping:

- **He might be teething. Signs include drooling, runny nose, rash on chin, red cheeks, rejecting breast or bottle, wanting to suck more, nappy rash**
- **He might be ill. Ear infections are common in babies because their Eustachian tubes are so small, but unfortunately they are incredibly painful, especially when he is lying down. He may seem fine when you hold him upright. If your baby seems to be crying in pain, has a fever, diarrhoea, reduced appetite, runny nose or any other worrying symptoms, ring your GP.**

'CORE NIGHT'
One idea which might appeal to you is the idea of a 'core night' – that is, the idea of identifying the first time your baby sleeps for a significant stretch of time during the night, and aiming to stretch this to gradually longer and longer periods by not feeding him if he wakes, but comforting him in other ways.[2] As time goes on, aim to make this core night a little longer, avoiding feeding him during these hours. Some parents find this works for them, although research suggests it's not necessarily particularly effective.[3]

'FOCUS FEEDING'
Another suggestion which some parents find works for them, is to create a 'focus feed' – usually just before they go to bed themselves

– where you try to get your baby to feed for a long time, to really fill up before bedtime. This can apply equally to breast- or bottle-feeding. Some parents 'top up' a breastfeed with a bottle of expressed milk or formula at this point, too.

However, recent research investigating whether focal feeds were effective in helping babies to sleep longer found that they did not help, mainly because parents were unwilling to implement them; the thought being that if the baby was asleep, they didn't want to wake him. So if you like the idea of a focus feed, try it, but be aware that there are no research studies to clarify whether this works or not.[4]

Changing Times

Even if you are happy with how your young baby sleeps, don't expect things to stay static. Over time, he will change, and you will need to be adaptable. Your six-month-old may happily sleep on his own, but when he reaches eight or fifteen months of age, and goes through a clingy phase as is usual at these ages, he might become afraid of being abandoned, and get distressed at awaking to a silent, empty bedroom. It's hard when your efforts to establish routines seem to be disappearing out of the window, but recognize what is happening for your baby, be sensitive to his needs, and adapt your routines as you both see fit.

Coping with Broken Nights

When you are expecting a baby, the thought of sleep-deprivation can fill you with terror. But remember:

- **Your body prepares you for broken nights during pregnancy.**
- **If you breastfeed, your hormones help you get back to sleep quickly.**

Helping Your Baby Stay Asleep 149 ♥

- Broken nights feel worse if you miss REM sleep. You can recover this with a good doze during the day. Make yourself lie down for an hour or so while your baby is sleeping.
- Take turns with your partner to get up for baby in the pre-dawn hours, when your body does most REM sleep.
- Go to bed really early, or have a lie-in, at least once a week, if you can, to 'catch up'.
- Don't expect too much of yourself in the early days.

Exercise for remaining mentally calm when your baby is screaming:

1. Take a deep breath. Imagine that it is bringing calmness with it.
2. Then imagine a picture of your baby smiling.
3. Focus all your thoughts on the smiling baby.
4. Smile back at him.
5. Feel your emotions beginning to change and calm as you smile.
6. Project the picture of the smiling baby on to the crying baby until his mood begins to change and he shares your smiley feelings.

— *Rosemary, mother of Nicholas and Sophie*

~ Times Change ~ Answer – 1985 ~

From Ferber, 'How to Solve Your Child's Sleep Problems' – quoted by James McKenna in La Leche League Great Britain News *May/June 2001*

22

All Change: Sleep and the Older Baby

~ Times change – does the advice stay the same? ~

*The conditions which kept life simple and natural 50 years ago
have largely changed; there is now more to stimulate the nervous
system and less opportunity for muscular development. One of the
most important reasons for this is the far greater proportion of
children who are reared in cities and large towns, shut away from
nature, free movement and play. Innocent children are becoming
miniature men and women before their time.*

Even if your young baby sleeps as you would like her to, don't expect
things to stay static. Once she starts toddling, good night-time habits
seem to fly out of the window!

The biggest change, as your baby becomes a toddler, is the need for
boundaries. Babies are happy to go along with everything you suggest,
but toddlers want to assert their independence, and quickly realize
that night-time is when they can really make an impact!

Bedtime Battles

You may think that having a battle putting your toddler to bed means she needs less sleep, but this is usually not true. Roughly speaking, at 18 months your baby still needs 12 hours a night and up to 2 hours during the day; by three years of age she will still need 12 hours at night but may have dropped the daytime sleep, although a quiet rest after lunch is good for recharging batteries.

A child who's not getting enough sleep will be grumpy, irritable and generally difficult. Many tired children become hyperactive; the more tired they are, the more manic and out of control they can seem. Sound familiar? If your child is cheerful and contented, alert and active, she may well be getting enough sleep, but if she's difficult during the day, then perhaps she's overtired.

DID YOU KNOW?
– No child is ever a perfect sleeper!

Most research will draw conclusions by taking samples of children of different ages at the same time and working out statistical averages. Few studies are longitudinal – that is, looking at the same children over time to see how they develop.

One study did look at the same 150 babies at ages 6, 12, 18 and 24 months. They found that 63 per cent of the children did not have sleeping difficulties at any age; however, for the rest, half the infants changed from having sleeping difficulties to not having sleeping difficulties, while the other half changed in the opposite direction.

So if a baby was not a good sleeper at 6 months, she might well sleep well at 12 and 18 months, while one who had been sleeping well at 6 months might start waking when she was older.

Only 5 per cent of the babies had sleeping difficulties at every age; instead, there is considerable variety in sleeping patterns at all ages.[1]

I WON'T GO TO BED!

Your toddler realizes that Mummy and Daddy stay up and have fun without her! Why should she go to bed? She's tired and out of sorts; she's bound to be unreasonable. She really wants you to be firm, to set boundaries calmly and with gentle persistence. Screaming at her to go to sleep will only work her up more.

If you haven't yet established a bedtime routine, now's really the time. Have a look back at pages 137–43 to find out why winding down, with the same sequence of calming events each night, helps your toddler feel secure and dozy. A suggested routine could be:

1 bath
2 milky drink
3 brush teeth
4 goodnight kiss downstairs for everyone
5 bedtime story in bed
6 kiss and cuddle, and both saying 'Night, night!'

Your routine needs to involve winding down, so obviously a wild romp with Daddy or an hour of TV is not ideal. Apart from that, it doesn't really matter what you choose to do; a bedtime routine is basically about keeping things predictable.

I DON'T WANT TO BE ALONE!

Many toddlers develop separation anxiety, and need extra reassurance before being left to settle down for the night. Watch out for this turning into a delaying tactic!

If you find that settling your toddler to bed is taking longer and longer:

- **Follow your routine of story, kisses and cuddles, plus lots of reassurance.**

- **Decide on a time-limit for settling your toddler, and stick to it firmly.**
- **Leave a night-light on or a lullaby tape playing after you leave.**

We've already looked at behaviour modification and leaving your child to cry. As we've seen, for babies this is probably inappropriate, but for a toddler who is really testing your boundaries, it might well work, as long as you feel you understand why your toddler is being difficult about bedtimes, and you are prepared to explain what you are doing.

HELP! I HAD A BAD DREAM!
It is no good telling your child it was 'just a bad dream'; to her it was real. Instead, respond to the nightmare at face value, doing whatever you think will reassure your child. For instance, if she says there was a monster, tell her you have sent it away and locked the door and now it can't get back in.

If she's having frequent nightmares, consider how much stimulation she gets late afternoon and early evening. If she watches TV, choose a soothing, calming video or, better still, read a gentle story. Keep a diary and see if you can detect a pattern to the nightmares. Do they happen on nursery days? Are they related to potty-training?

OTHER NIGHT-WAKING
Children who always fall asleep with a parent in the room will feel abandoned if they wake in the night to find themselves alone. To avoid night terrors, make sure your toddler is managing to fall asleep on her own.

Sleep Associations

Some toddlers won't sleep through the night if they've learned that something nice – like food or a long cuddle – happens if they wake up. Start cutting any 'night treats' down. Instead of rushing in to cuddle her, reassure your child from the doorway of her bedroom. A toddler will not need feeding in the night, but may be thirsty; substitute water for middle-of-the-night milky drinks – water is not really worth waking up for, a milk or juice drink is.

BEDROOM VERSUS PLAYROOM

A bedroom is your child's personal space, and it is tempting to keep all her toys in there – if only to keep the rest of the house feeling sane. But if a bedroom is too stimulating, your child will find it hard to get to sleep or to stay asleep. Think about keeping toys in another part of the house, or tidying them away in large, plain cupboards so your toddler can't see them from her cot.

Is it Morning Yet?

What can you do with a child who wakes bright as a button, but too early? All of us experience shallow sleep in the early hours, but we grown-ups are used to falling asleep again. Your baby is capable, but if she's over-stimulated, she will force herself to stay awake. Consider:

- **Is she getting too much stimulation in the day, so she has too much to think about in the early hours?**
- **Is her bedroom too stimulating?**
- **Perhaps her bedroom needs to be darker?**

If she's a persistent early bird, you could put a few restful toys, like teddies or soft books, in her cot to play with when she wakes so she will be content until you are ready to face the day!

All Change: Sleep and the Older Baby 155

REWARDS

It is often better to use positive rewards with a toddler than punishment. For a reward to be effective, it has to be meaningful and understandable. A two-year-old will not be able to cope with, 'If you stay in bed every night this week, we will take you out at the weekend' – it's all just too big. But 'If you stay in bed in the morning and play quietly until Mummy comes in to see you, you can have a comic book when we go shopping in the morning' is just about do-able.

Toddlers are capable of delayed gratification, but their time scale is still short, so rewards need to be fairly immediate. The other important thing about rewards is that you have to be willing to withhold them if they are not deserved! And don't offer, as a reward, something you were intending to do anyway.

With older children, star charts can be effective. One star for getting into bed by 7 p.m., another for staying in bed until 7 a.m., and so on, adding up over a week to a reward for 10 stars, say, at the end of the week.

If they 'fail' on occasion, don't berate them – you can even sympathize with them: 'What a shame, no star today! Never mind, I'm sure you can manage one tonight!'

Some Other Things to Remember

- **Don't sent your children to bed for being naughty; that way bed becomes associated with unpleasant things.**
- **Some children are better sleepers than others – don't be tempted to compare your children with your friends' children.**
- **If you are overtired it's harder to be consistent, and consistency is really important with toddlers! Make sure you**

get enough sleep yourself; if necessary, lie down after lunch when she does if you can.

- Although it seems to go against logic, children who are tired tend to become hyperactive, so if your child is bouncing off the wall, don't assume she doesn't need to go to bed!
- A tired and irritable child is harder to deal with, so try to pre-empt this by starting the bedtime routine *before* she gets grouchy.
- Don't let her sleep too late or too long in the afternoon, unless you want her to stay up all evening.

James, who is 20 months, has always slept with us, and hardly ever fully wakes at night. When he was little he used to just snuffle around and latch on. If you are waking in the night, your sleep patterns coincide with your baby's, so you just gradually wake up with them. When they are in a cot you can't be so in touch, you don't hear them snuffling around. The first thing you hear is crying and that means you have to wake up quickly and they are already awake.

– *Margaret, mother of James*

~ Times Change ~ Answer – 1899 ~

Dr Hall and Dr Holt in the welcoming address to the third annual convention of the National Congress of Mothers in Washington DC, mid-February 1899.

From The Wilson Quarterly *(Winter 1999)*

23

Who Sleeps Where?

~ Times change – does the advice stay the same? ~

*There is not anything in nature which is more immediately
calculated to subvert health, strength, love, esteem and indeed
everything that is desirable in the married state than that odious,
most indelicate and most hurtful custom of man and wife
continually pigging together in one and the same bed. Nothing is
more unwise or unnatural than for a man and woman to sleep,
snore and do everything else that is indelicate together, three
hundred and sixty five times a year.*

Most people do not sleep alone. Wherever and whenever you look,
throughout human society, bed-sharing is the norm. Even today in
the West, the majority of people share a bed with someone else.
Adults sleep together not just for sex; we all know how pleasant it is
to snuggle up next to another body in the middle of the night. Why
then, is there such a taboo against having children in the bed or even
the bedroom?

Until the 18th century in this country, communal sleeping was normal; often several people would sleep together – which is why beds from these times are so enormous.[1] Beds were for sex and sleeping, but also for chatting, entertaining and keeping warm, and several generations of a family, as well as visitors and friends, would tuck up under the covers for the night.

Once the Industrial Revolution happened, and people started to work away from home, the extended family began to disperse, and enormous beds became less common. Only the immediate family of parents and children would sleep together. In the UK babies still slept with their mothers or nurses as a matter of course.

However, as people began to understand a bit more about germs, a reluctance to bed-share took hold, and early in the 20th century not only were babies banished to the nursery, married couples also slept in twin beds to avoid spreading germs. Later in the century we couples decided to risk it, and moved back into the double bed, germs and all, but somehow our babies were still left in the cold, expected to move from the womb, a world where noise and touch were constant, to a dark and silent nursery.

Another reason to leave babies in the nursery was that the notion of 'romantic love' and the importance of the husband-wife relationship were taking hold, and this meant baby took second place. It was also thought that a physical distance in particular between father and children would help father display moral authority and dispense religious training.[2]

Bed-sharing – Fashion or Necessity?

We now tend to view sharing a bed with a baby as either a 'bad thing' or perhaps as a 'consumer choice'. Both viewpoints ignore the fact that babies have evolved over millions of years to sleep with other human beings.

But many practices, which have been normal for human beings over the millions of years of our development, have now been abandoned. The argument goes that we now lead such totally different lifestyles to our ancestors, bed-sharing is no longer appropriate or sensible. After all, we've got to get up for work in the morning!

Sharing – Does It Disturb Your Sleep?

One study filmed partners sleeping together and found that they usually change position simultaneously (a sleeping pattern called *synchrony*) without being aware of it. People move around more when sleeping with a partner than when sleeping alone, yet most will say they sleep better when their partner is present.[3]

Is it any different for mothers and babies, or even parents and babies? No, it's not. When mother and baby bed-sharing has been studied in the laboratory, synchrony is also seen; mother and baby tune in to each other, and their cycles of arousal and sleep come together. So although the research shows that bed-sharing mothers wake more often, they actually spend just as much time asleep over-all as mothers whose babies sleep in another room, and tend to feel less disturbed, for two reasons:

1 As mother and baby tune into each other, they both wake at the end of their cycle, when arousal would happen naturally. Neither wakes fully and the baby doesn't cry; he attracts his mother's attention with arm and body movements.[4]

2 If your baby sleeps in a separate room and wakes alone, he has to cry to attract your attention, and in the process, will get agitated and upset.[5] In the meantime, you have to get out of bed to

respond to your baby, so both of you wake up fully, and thus it takes longer for both of you to get back to sleep again. In addition, breastfeeding babies will not feed as effectively if they are already crying and upset, so they will need to wake again sooner.

Sleeping When You Have a New Baby

Pregnancy prepares women for a different sleeping pattern; pregnant women have less deep, slow-wave sleep – down to about 5 per cent compared with 25 per cent when not pregnant. Instead, there is more REM sleep. Women often have far more vivid dreams during pregnancy; perhaps this is because they have more time to dream. Perhaps this change is part of the process of fitting mother's and baby's sleep cycles together, because babies under four months have higher REM sleep and no deep sleep.

Even mothers who choose to sleep apart from their babies do not in fact sleep deeply; they do not often descend into Stage-four deep sleep because they wish to be able to hear their baby cry.[6]

As we will see in the next chapter, the research into SIDs suggests that co-sleeping (meaning in the same bed or in the same room) is far safer for a baby under six months. In addition, research suggests that co-sleeping is better for breastfeeding in that bed-sharing mothers and babies carry on breastfeeding for longer than mothers and babies who sleep separately.[7]

When Is Co-sleeping Appropriate?

Our society believes that it is better for babies to sleep alone, and that separate sleeping encourages independence, but in fact there is no research evidence to suggest that babies who sleep on their own are less dependent on their parents.

Others suggest that having a baby in the bed will prevent you sleeping properly, or even create marital discord by inhibiting your sex life! As we have seen, sharing a bed with anyone we are used to having there is not disrupting, and may even help us sleep. As to the sex life argument; I wonder how many couples with a very young baby are actually at it all night? Is spontaneous, hours-long sex the norm, or is it more likely that sex is 'on hold for the time being', with the odd quickie happening at a prearranged, pre-negotiated time?

Many surveys of postnatal sex lives, even allowing for probable exaggeration in this department, suggest that couples take a long time to get back to anything like 'normality', and while this has everything to do with the arrival of the baby, which room or bed he is in has little to do with it.

The short answer is, it's better to sleep with your baby; whether in the same room or the same bed is up to you. Wherever your baby sleeps, make sure he's safe – as per guidelines in the next chapter. If you are considering bed-sharing, make sure that you and your partner agree about this in the rational light of day rather than at 3 a.m.!

However, don't feel that early co-sleeping or occasional bed-sharing means that you will never have your bed to yourselves again. As Deborah Jackson puts it, 'It would be a poor show if we only started things which we did not have to finish. Our babies would never wear nappies or be breastfed at all.'[10]

OVERLAYING

For many parents, the idea of bed-sharing raises the fear of 'overlaying'. In fact, for a long time the two terms – cot death and overlaying – were synonymous, but this was at a time when all babies slept with parents. Any unexplained death was simply referred to as overlaying, whether the baby was actually smothered by another person or not. In fact, observations in laboratories suggest that mothers in particular are always very aware of where their babies are at all times, unless drugged or extremely tired.

MOVING ON

As to when you should move your baby into his own room, this is where opinion, politics and prejudice really start to muddy the waters. The biggest study ever into cot death – the CESDI study – concluded that sharing a bedroom for the first six months cuts the risk of cot death.[11] But some people move their babies earlier; some continue to co-sleep for far longer. There is no real answer – it is down to you, your partner and your baby when he should move out. In the current climate, people who choose to sleep with an older child will, unfortunately, not suffer from a lack of other people's opinions! Often the baby who knows he is welcome into his parents' bed is, ironically, less likely to need it![12]

However, it is probably best *not* to move your baby when:

- **He is likely to be going through a stage of having
  separation anxiety, anyway – at around 8 months, then
  again at 2 years.**

- Other big changes are happening – like moving house or having another baby. Move him several weeks before or after, so that only one unsettling event happens at a time.
- You are returning to work. Many working mothers like co-sleeping, as the physical closeness makes up for the daytime separation. If that's not for you, move your baby well before you return to work.
- Having your baby in another room would make you feel anxious. Parents get separation anxiety, too!

A Smooth Transition

There are several ways of easing the transition from your room to his.

- Do it in stages, so that first he goes in a cot by the side of the bed, then the cot moves across the room, and finally it moves into his own room.
- Some parents co-sleep in the baby's room for a little while, to smooth the transition.
- Another way to do it gradually is to have some of the night together and some alone; perhaps moving him back into his cot when he's asleep, and then praising him in the morning for the time he spent alone.
- Set up the monitor the wrong way round (so he can hear you breathing).
- Put something that smells of you in his cot – a nightie or a breastpad.
- Heat his cot with a hot water bottle – but remember to remove it *before* he gets in.
- Use the cot during the day for some pleasant time – reading stories or quiet play, so it feels like a good place to be.
- When moving an older child, make it a special event! Involve him in choosing bedcovers or a new night-time companion.

- If you are moving a much older child, one who is already talking, you can use positive reinforcement, such as star charts and rewards – see pages 156–7 for more about behaviour training techniques.

DID YOU KNOW?
– You have to feel good about it!
Researchers in North America investigated co-sleeping in different communities. Although advice there is generally against bed-sharing, in practice (as here in the UK) many parents do bed-share: nearly a third of the white families and three-quarters of black families interviewed routinely bed-shared.

For the white families, those who were co-sleeping had more bedtime struggles and more night-waking than those who slept separately, but all white families rated night-waking as having a negative impact on their own sleep.

The black families had similar levels of bedtime struggles and night-waking, but for those who co-slept, the night-waking was not described as disruptive. So even though more black families co-slept, fewer of them saw night-waking as disruptive.

The conclusion? Co-sleeping has different meanings and associations for different people – if you think it's OK, then probably it will feel OK.[13]

For night-time crying we found co-sleeping was the only thing that really worked. In the very early days with our first baby, when we were worried about squashing her, we slept with the Moses basket in the bed between us. With my second I find that the best way to get him to sleep (again, as we are worried about squashing him) is to lie him in our bed but on the mattress from his Moses basket, feed and cuddle him until he falls asleep, then transfer him and mattress together back into the basket.

– Hayley, mother of Elizabeth and Edward

~ Times change ~ Answer – 1783 ~

From Dr James Graham, 'A lecture on the Generation, Increase and Improvement of the Human Species', in Paul Martin, Counting Sheep *(HarperCollins, 2001)*

24

Sleeping Safely

~ Times change – does the advice stay the same? ~

Advert for twin beds: 'Never breathe the breath of another.'

Probably one of the worst things that can happen to a new family is to have their much-loved baby die suddenly and unexpectedly. The leading cause of death[1] in new babies is Sudden Infant Death Syndrome (SIDS), also known as cot death.

In 1992, the 'Back to Sleep' campaign was launched, encouraging parents to place their babies to sleep on their backs. As a result, the SIDS rate fell by 70 per cent.[2] However, seven babies still die each week from cot death in the UK alone. Why is this, and what can you, as a parent, do to minimize the risk for your baby?

Which Babies Are at Risk?

Eighty-six per cent of SIDS victims die before they reach six months of age, and the greatest numbers of deaths occur around age two to three months; rarely does cot death happen after 12 months of age (3.7 per cent of all cot deaths).

Boys die more frequently than girls (60 per cent of all cot deaths), and low birth-weight is also a risk factor. In addition, about 18 per cent of all SIDS deaths involve premature infants.[3] Most babies are found dead in their cots (hence the name), though babies have died in other places, too.

Causes of Cot Death

There isn't just one reason for babies to die suddenly and unexpectedly. It may even be that for each baby, the reason is different; some factors may work together, while some infants are more vulnerable in certain ways than others.

First Principles – Back to Sleep

Why is the supine position so important?

Over 20 years ago, researchers noticed that newborn babies who were sleeping on their backs were twice as active and woke more often than babies who slept on their stomachs. As the goal was, and still is, to encourage babies to sleep through the night, books began to suggest that babies be placed on their tummies to sleep;[4] tragically, however, this has since been found to be the main cause of cot death.

There are lots of reasons why prone sleeping might be dangerous for newborn babies. It may be that they end up breathing their own exhaled carbon dioxide, especially if they are trapped under thick blankets.[5] Perhaps breathing is less easy when face-down, simply because this position restricts the movement of the chest. One group of researchers suggested that between 28 and 52 per cent of SIDS victims found face-down might have actually suffocated.[6]

Remember – put your baby 'Back to Sleep'

Smoking

For babies who are safely sleeping on their backs, maternal smoking, particularly in pregnancy, is the next major risk. A recent study found that babies whose mothers had smoked during pregnancy were almost five times as likely to die compared with the babies of non-smokers. It is less clear whether passive smoking has an effect, but where Father smokes and Mother doesn't, the risk for baby increases 1.4 times over having two non-smoking parents.[7]

Don't let people smoke near your baby. Don't sleep with your baby if you smoke.

Good Practice – Breastfeeding

Breastfeeding does reduce the risk of cot death, though the effect is not as great as the correct sleeping position.[8] The suggestion that breastfeeding helps prevent cot death has not been widely publicized in the UK, as it is felt that other factors confuse the picture. For instance, breastfeeding mothers and babies are more likely to bed-share than bottle-feeding mother and babies, and, as we shall see, where your baby sleeps is also important.

Breastfeeding seems to give your baby additional protection against cot death.

Over-heating

It used to be thought that cot death was caused by overheating; however, since babies have been placed on their backs to sleep, this is felt to be less of an issue,[11] although a few babies do still die from overheating.[12] If your baby is sleeping on her own, keep her room at a temperature of between 16-20°C, and use one or more layers of light blankets, not a duvet, quilt or pillow.[13]

Avoid overheating your baby.

Using Old Mattresses

In the early 1990s there were media reports that Cot Death may have been associated with second-hand mattresses. Again, this is a factor, but the most recent research suggests it only has an effect if the mattress came from another household; there does not seem to be an increased risk if the mattress was used before by your baby's sibling, so you don't need to buy a new mattress for every baby.[14]

It is important to make sure that the mattress fits the cot well and that it is thoroughly clean, which is easier if it is covered with PVC or other waterproof cover.[15]

Use a new mattress for your family.

SIDS – An Arousal Deficit?

The most recent research into SIDS has focused on babies' ability to control their breathing and arousal during sleep.[16]

The brain stem controls our being awake, as well as time spent in the different sleep stages, and one particular area may be responsible for keeping oxygen and carbon dioxide levels balanced. Post-mortems on SIDS victims have suggested that some babies have deficits in this area of the brain, so that perhaps they cannot rouse themselves after particularly long breathing pauses.

Premature and/or low birth-weight infants are at particular risk of SIDS; so, it also seems, are babies who have experienced one or more 'apparent life-threatening events' (ALTE) defined as loss of muscle tone accompanied by gasping or choking, listlessness, colour changes, or stopping breathing. Approximately 6 per cent of infants who experience an ALTE die from SIDS. Perhaps vulnerable babies have problems with arousal and regulating their breathing.

HOW USEFUL IS A MONITOR?

It's fine to use a simple monitor that allows you to listen to your baby when you are out of the room. The more expensive and elaborate monitors, which electronically monitor the baby's breathing and movement, are really best for babies who are identified as at particular risk, and your paediatrician will recommend one to you in those circumstances.

Research indicates that elaborate monitors make parents more stressed, unless they have had intensive guidance and counselling in their proper use.[17]

Co-sleeping as Protection Against SIDS

The most recent and most comprehensive research into Cot Death in this country has concluded that sharing a room with a parent halves the risk of death.[18] The study also found that bed-sharing was fine when certain precautions are met – see the safe sleeping suggestions at the end of this chapter.

A newborn baby has a natural gasping reflex when in danger of suffocation, but this reflex is lost after a few weeks and thereafter the baby depends to some extent on adults to regulate her breathing.[19]

Research has found that when mothers and babies sleep together, they face each other, close enough to inhale each other's carbon dioxide, suggesting that perhaps the mother is stimulating the baby to breathe more regularly.[20]

In Asia, where bed-sharing is the norm, SIDS rates are very low. Interestingly, when Asian families emigrate to the West, they still have low SIDS rate, though as they live here longer the rates get higher, perhaps because they start to adopt Western cultural norms and so sleep apart from their babies.[21]

James McKenna, Professor of Anthropology and Director of the Mother-Baby Behavioural Sleep Laboratory at the University of Notre Dame in Indiana, has pioneered research into bed-sharing, and he suggests that babies with impaired arousal mechanisms benefit from bed-sharing as they spend less time in deep sleep. He found that bed-sharing mothers lean over and inspect their babies six to ten times during the night, thus providing more arousal practice,[22-] as well as prolonging the duration of these arousals.[23]

> *It's safest to share your room with your baby for at least the first six months, and bed-sharing is fine if it's done safely.*

Other Regulatory Mechanisms

Deborah Jackson, author of *Three in a Bed*, points out that babies have to change the way they breathe in order to speak, with breathing slowing from 87 to around 47 breaths per minute, and the time these changes are happening – between two and four months of age – are also the time when a baby is most susceptible to SIDS.[24]

Babies thrive with skin-to-skin contact, which research has shown helps stabilize heart rates, increases body temperature, and reduces sleep apnoeas and crying.[25]

James McKenna points out that, for ape babies, short-term separation from their mothers has serious consequences for their physiology, resulting in reduced skin temperature, irregular heart beats, depressed immune responses, increased stress and even reduced antibodies in the blood.

He and his research team were the first to measure electrophysiological differences between solitary sleeping and bed-sharing mother-baby pairs. Contrary to conventional thinking, bed-sharing infants breathe better, sleep more, feed better and maintain more stable body temperatures.[26]

Safe Bed-sharing

- You need to make sure your baby can't fall out of bed. One way is to push your bed against the wall, but it can be difficult ensuring there's no gap between the wall and the base of the bed or the mattress. It might be better to use a guardrail; a plastic mesh is probably safer than one with slats. Again, make sure it's flush against the side of your mattress, so your baby can't slip into a gap. You can also now buy sidecar cots where the side drops down and the cot mattress can be raised to be on the same level as your bed.
- Don't put your baby to sleep alone in an adult bed.
- If there are other children in the bed, don't let them sleep next to the baby.
- Use as big a bed as possible.
- Avoid large pillows or cushions, and don't sleep with your baby on a couch or water bed, as these surfaces are too soft. Surfaces should be firm.
- It's sensible to avoid wearing necklaces and clothes with string ties when you sleep with your baby.
- Be aware of overheating – your baby will need fewer clothes than if she were sleeping alone.

> **DID YOU KNOW?**
> **– Back to sleep is safer for your baby, but it's bad news for your sleep!**
>
> Although it is safer for babies to sleep on their backs, in fact they awake more easily from this position. When mothers and babies bed-share, the babies are always placed on their backs, as this makes it easier for the baby to breastfeed. McKenna suggests that babies who sleep on their own are more at risk of being placed prone.[27] He noticed that when mothers were bed-sharing they always placed the babies on their backs, but the same mothers would sometimes place the babies prone when sleeping alone.[28]

- Make sure that duvet or pillows cannot cover your baby's head. It is better to use lightweight blankets, rather than an adult duvet.

WHEN NOT TO SHARE
- If you or your partner are smokers.
- If you have been drinking or taking drugs (this includes prescribed drugs such as sedatives or strong painkillers).
- If you are extremely tired.

Safety in the Cot

- Don't use an old cot or old mattress – make sure it conforms to current British Safety Standards.
- Make sure the mattress fits without any gaps.
- It's best not to use cot bumpers, but if you do, there should be plenty (at least six) ties, and each of these should be no longer than six inches.
- Put your baby on her back to sleep.
- Don't use pillows or soft bedding which could pose a risk of suffocation.
- Use blankets rather than a duvet for babies less than a year old; tuck the covers in firmly and make the cot up from the bottom – so your baby sleeps 'feet to foot'.
- Avoid overheating the room or overdressing your baby.
- When your baby learns to sit, lower the mattress level so that she cannot climb out, and remove cot bumpers.
- Hang mobiles well out of reach, and remove them when your baby can sit up.

Effie had dreadful colic from about 10 weeks. Heartrending, endless crying all evening, just when you are most unable to cope. She was only soothed by a warm bath, which quietened her completely, but as soon as she was lifted out the crying started again; but even 20 minutes of peace was a sanity-saver.

All my babies were restive in the evening and were difficult to settle. Our best solution was to buy a baby backpack and Nigel would load them in and take them for a fast, purposeful walk around the streets. In less than 10 minutes they were deeply enough asleep to be gently tipped from the backpack into bed.

– Belinda, mother of Martha, Effie and Kitty

~ Times Change ~ Answer – 1893 ~

Scrivener's Magazine *in Paul Martin*, Counting Sheep (*HarperCollins, 2001*)

25

Putting it All Together: What's Going to Work for You?

~ Times change – does the advice stay the same? ~
To sleep, perchance to dream ...

One of the worst things you can do to someone is to prevent them falling asleep. Amnesty International finds that more than half of the torture victims they interview have been deprived of sleep for at least 24 hours. Sleep deprivation helps in brainwashing; it also leads to irritability, memory lapses, hallucinations; you lose the ability to string sentences together or to concentrate. If it goes on long enough, it can be fatal: according to legend, King Perseus of Macedonia was put to death by being prevented from sleeping, one of the worst ways to die.[1]

Scary stuff? If you are reading this book while you're expecting with your first baby, you probably already have strong ideas about how, where and when your baby will sleep, and your partner will too. Will you both agree, though?

The Cyclical Nature of Parenting Ideas

As you may have noticed from the quotes at the beginning of each chapter, there has never been a shortage of advice for new parents, and each generation will encounter a new trend, fad – call it what you will. All that we can be sure of is that every generation seems keen to ignore the advice of the previous generation, often choosing to do completely the opposite. The other sure fact is that everyone has a strong opinion about babies and sleep.

Influences

How you will feel about the issue of responding to your baby, particularly at night, may well be influenced by how you were treated as a baby yourself. Were you 'left to cry'? If you were, and if you can remember this, it may be that for you the idea of your baby crying, even for a couple of minutes, is abhorrent.

There is a chance, of course, that if your partner is of similar age, background and culture, his parents may have read the same books as your parents, and he may therefore have had a similar upbringing. There is also the possibility that he will feel the same as you do.

On the other hand, perhaps your partner spent the night in his parents' bed, and his memories are of being secure, warm and nurtured. Perhaps he would like to offer this experience to his own baby, but then again, having had his needs met, he may feel less distressed by his baby's cries and may be more willing to follow advice which suggests leaving babies to cry.

Both of these approaches – leaving a baby to cry, never letting a baby cry – have points in their favour, depending on the age of the baby, but neither are, in themselves, 'right' or 'wrong'. But they will evoke a strong reaction in both of you, and it's important for your relationship that you and your partner know what you are doing and why. Try to discuss how you feel about sleep issues when you are both alert and functioning, rather than at 2 a.m. when all you want to do is to sleep!

It is also worth bearing in mind that as babies have different sleep patterns at each age in their first year, it would make no sense to expect the same behaviour at each stage, nor would it make any sense to use the same strategy for a newborn baby as you would use for a six-month-old, or even a six-year-old.

The Psychoanalytic Perspective

Dilys Daws is a psychotherapist who works at the Tavistock Institute in London, helping parents who have children with sleep difficulties. She views sleep difficulties as the result of a failure to resolve issues about the relationship between the infant and parents, in particular feelings about separation.

'The setting up of a baby's sleep-wake rhythms is influenced by interaction between parent and baby,' she says.

Her therapeutic work is designed to help parents and baby be better able to deal with separation. She talks about the ability to let go of each other emotionally, in order to go to sleep.

'A problem could be considered to exist when the baby's reason for waking is not understood, when the parent feels the waking up is not reasonable, or when an apparent habit has passed but the baby continues to wake as a fixed habit. All these can be thought of in terms of how parents and infant are getting on with each other in their managing of the baby's physiological state.'[2]

Rather than get hung up about what other people tell you 'ought' to happen, perhaps you could just think about what you and your family want. For instance, if you are breastfeeding at night and finding it OK, then you might be content to wait until your baby seems ready to sleep for longer. If, however, you feel like a zombie and that sleep-deprivation is a form of torture, then it is time to cut down on night-feeding!

Conclusions: Whose Problem Is It?

While I have suggested ways of helping your baby to settle and to sleep, it is worth taking time at this point to consider, what is a sleep problem as far as you are concerned? And why is it a problem? Are you trying to do what other people tell you to do? Remember that one person's problem is another person's solution.

Another important fact about raising children is that today's solution works today, but it may

**DID YOU KNOW?
– Everyone's sleeping arrangements are unique!**
Helen Ball's latest research has been looking at bed-sharing twins, and generally if twins share the same cot, they stay in their parents' room for much longer, probably because it is physically easier to keep one cot in the room than two. Families used one of the following positions:

– side-by-side lengthways
– head-to-head lengthways
– foot-to-foot lengthways
– side-by-side widthways
– diagonally with head in the corner, feet in the middle for one twin, and head in the middle, feet in the corner for the other.

If twins were side-by-side lengthways, they generally had identical sleep patterns; if one did wake and cry it did not disturb the other, nor did they overheat in comparison to the nights they spent separately.[3]

no longer be appropriate tomorrow. You might not be able to let your six-year-old wander around the streets on her own during the day, but you should probably allow your 16-year-old to do so. Potty-training in our society might not work for a two-week-old baby or a two-month-old baby, but it may well work for a two-year-old baby.

Why would strategies for comforting your baby, or getting her to sleep, be any different? If you choose to sleep with your two-week-old baby, this does not mean that you will be forced to sleep with your two-year-old baby or even your 20-year-old offspring. It is a good idea to let a teenager cry it out; toddlers also need to learn that they can't have everything they want, but is this an appropriate way to handle a new baby?

Remember, too, if you are reading this during pregnancy, that once your baby is born and you have a third personality to consider, the ideas you hold dearly now may completely change. All this is fine. Welcome to the ever-changing, ever-flexible world of parenting!

For the first two and a half months, my daughter cried when I put her down; feeding or carrying her seemed to be the only ways of calming her. At this stage I couldn't work out why she was crying, and just used to try feeding her first, walking around with her, changing her or putting her down if that failed. I used a sling carrier a lot – whenever we went out, for feeding at times, and to do the vacuuming!

Suddenly, when she was about 10 or 11 weeks old, she started to sort out her own routine and enjoy time separated from me, lying under the play-gym or in her bouncy chair.

Until then she had slept in a carrycot in our bedroom, but as she had dropped to only one night-time feed I started to gradually move her into the cot in her own room. Initially, I would put her down in her big cot, wake her around 10:30 p.m. for a feed, and then settle her in the carrycot in our bedroom as we went to bed. As she seemed very happy in her cot and I knew I'd hear her when she woke, at about four months I moved her fully to the cot, at least partly because she had outgrown the carrycot and was very noisy snuffling around at night.

– Carol, mother to Autumn

Carol and Autumn make for a good way of rounding off this book. For Carol, the first 10 weeks were spent responding closely to Autumn's need for physical comfort, as she gradually adapted to the world outside her mother's body. As Carol's baby learned that she was safe, and could count on her mother being there for her, she was able to start enjoying time being separate, discovering new experiences through play, which is how babies learn. Autumn's need for her mother at night also began to lessen, and she began to sleep for longer continuous periods. At around four months, her mother's own need for a good night's sleep then took precedence, and Autumn was moved into her cot.

All children are unique – yours is unlikely to follow the same pattern – but Carol's experience is shown here as an example; it's one parent's way of dealing with her baby's changing needs. Being a parent is all about learning to trust your gut feelings, finding out what works best, not just for your child, but for you too; being open to change; and staying flexible and reponsive – as I hope this book has made clear.

~ Times change ~ Answer – 1602 ~

From Shakespeare's Hamlet

Cows' Milk-free Diet for Breastfeeding Mothers

Written by Elaine Antcliff BA SRD for the Breastfeeding Counsellor's Panel of the National Childbirth Trust.

> *This diet sheet has been written primarily for breastfeeding mothers whose babies are suffering from colic. However, there are many possible explanations for colic; sensitivity to cows' milk in the mother's diet is but one.*

Breastfed babies with eczema may also benefit from their mother avoiding cows' milk.

At first, keep strictly to this diet for two weeks, as some babies take this long to respond. If there is no change in your baby by the end of this time, it is unlikely that continuing the diet will have any benefit.

A strict cows' milk-free diet involves cutting out cows' milk and all its products, along with any manufactured products that also contain cows' milk. This means avoiding any kind of cows' milk whether it is whole, semi-skimmed, skimmed, dried, evaporated or condensed, and also avoiding cheese, yoghurt, cream, ice-cream, butter and margarine.

Check all manufactured products for the following: Milk, milk products, non-fat milk solids, skimmed milk, cream, artificial cream, cheese, yoghurt, butter, margarine, milk sugar, lactose, whey, hydrolysed whey sugar, casein, caseinate and hydrolysed casein.

This may appear to be a vast list, but you soon get used to checking ingredients and if you stick to fresh foods as much as possible the diet will be easier.

Milk-free Margarines

The majority of margarines contain milk. A margarine made from pure vegetable fat (such as Tomor, Granose or Vitaquell) is suitable. Some low-fat spreads and pure soya margarines are also suitable, but check ingredients carefully as manufactured products change frequently.

Adequate Energy Intake

Whilst breastfeeding, your diet is very important. You need to eat well to feel fit while breastfeeding. Cutting out cows' milk and all its products may mean you are reducing your energy intake quite substantially, especially if you ate a lot of cheese previously. You will, therefore, have to make these up by eating more of other foods.

Drinking water whenever you feel thirsty is important, too.

Calcium

A cows' milk-free diet can be very low in calcium. Breastfeeding mothers need extra calcium (1,200 mg per day) to ensure that their baby gets sufficient for his/her bones and teeth and to protect themselves from osteoporosis.

CALCIUM EXCHANGE LIST

The following 'exchange list' will help you. Each portion contains 100 mg calcium. Try to include at least eight exchanges per day.

Fish

Sardines (tinned including bones)	20 gm
Salmon (tinned including bones)	20 gm
Whitebait (fried)	5 gm
Pilchards (tinned including bones)	30 gm
Sprats (fried)	15 gm
Shrimp	30 gm
Prawns	70 gm

Bread

White bread	105 gm
Wholemeal bread	90 gm

(This is only true for certain brands of wholemeal bread. Check the nutritional information on the wrapper.)

Fruit

Apricots (dried or fresh)	105 gm
Blackberries (fresh)	165 gm
Blackcurrants (fresh)	180 gm
Figs (dried or fresh)	40 gm
Oranges (fresh – no peel)	255 gm
Rhubarb (fresh)	105 gm

(Some fruit juices now contain added calcium – for example, Tropicana pure premium. Try to drink 122 mg/100 ml a day.)

Vegetables

Broccoli tops (uncooked)	105 gm
Savoy cabbage (uncooked)	135 gm
Spinach (boiled)	15 gm
Spring greens (boiled)	120 gm
Watercress (raw)	45 gm
Baked beans (in tomato sauce)	230 gm
Red kidney beans (raw weight – ensure that they are cooked thoroughly)	75 gm

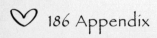

Sesame Seeds

Whole, without skins   15 gm

Without skins   90 gm

(Dark-coloured tahini – as made by Sunwheel foods, for example –
is therefore richer in calcium than a lighter-coloured one.)

Most of the fruits and vegetables are given as a raw weight, but this
does not mean that they have to be eaten raw. Once weighed, you
can cook them if you wish.

If you live in a hard-water area, approximately 850 ml of tap water
will give you 100 mg of calcium. Some bottled waters now contain
added calcium, such as DanoneActiv, which has 300 mg/litre.

CALCIUM SUPPLEMENTS

If you are unable to obtain enough calcium from your food, you will
need to take a calcium supplement. There are several brands available, including chewable tablets and effervescent soluble ones that
can be taken in a drink.

MILK SUBSTITUTES

Goats' milk may be used instead of cows' milk: it contains a different
type of protein, but similar amounts of calcium. Goats' milk cheese
and yoghurt may also be used.

Liquid soya milks, available in supermarkets and health food shops,
can be very low in calcium so are not a replacement for cows' milk
nutritionally. Make sure you choose one that is fortified with calcium. Even if you do not like the taste of soya milk, it makes very
palatable custard and 'milk' puddings.

Vitamin D

Vitamin D is very important, as it helps calcium to be absorbed. It is found mainly in margarines, low-fat spreads and oily fish. During the summer months, most people *get all* they need when their skin is exposed to sunlight. Some calcium supplements contain added vitamin D.

Reintroducing Cows' Milk

If you find that the diet helps, it may be worth continuing for a few weeks or months. Try drinking a glass of milk about once a month to see if there is any effect on your baby. If there is, continue with a strict cows' milk-free diet. If not, the diet may not be necessary, although some mothers find large amounts of milk or cheese may affect their baby.

Supplementary Feeds

Try to ensure your baby has breastmilk only. It is a good idea to express some and freeze it for emergencies. It will keep three months in the freezer. However, if you do give your baby a supplement, it is best to use modified infant soya milk or a hypoallergenic infant formula.

Please note that goats' milk is not suitable for babies.

Weaning

When your baby is ready for solids, you must be careful not to give baby foods containing cows' milk or its products. Check all ingredients carefully.

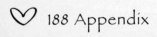

Link with Colic, Eczema and Food Intolerance

Some babies who suffer from colic or eczema also suffer from food intolerance. It is wise to seek further help from your GP, who will refer you to a paediatrician to enable a specific diagnosis to be made. As a result of this referral you should then receive appropriate dietary advice from a paediatric dietitian, and an approved soya or hypoallergenic milk formula will be prescribed for your baby if necessary.

References

Your Baby from Birth to Toddlerhood

1. WHY DO BABIES CRY?

1 Desmond Morris, *Babywatching* (Jonathan Cape, 1991)
2 Dr Harvey Karp, *The Happiest Baby on the Block* (Penguin/Michael Joseph, 2002)
3 *Ibid.*
4 Sheila Kitzinger, *Crying Baby* (Penguin, 1990)
5 Barry Lester, *et al.*, 'Developmental outcome as a function of the goodness of fit between the infant's cry characteristics and the mother's perception of her infant's cry', *Pediatrics* 95.4 (April 1995): 516–21
6 Quotes taken from the website for Brown Alumni Magazine (Jan/Feb 1999) –http://www.brown.edu/Administration/Brown_Alumni_Magazine/99/1-99/features/crying
7 T Berry Brazelton and J Kevin Nugent, *Neonatal Behavioural Assessment Scale* (3rd edn; MacKeith Press, 1995; distributed by Cambridge University Press)

2. GETTING USED TO THE WORLD: THE FIRST SIX WEEKS

1 Tine Thevenin, *Mothering and Fathering: The Gender Differences in Child Rearing* (Avery Publishing, 1993)
2 Rene Spitz, as cited in Lise Elliot, *Early Intelligence* (Penguin, 1999)

3. LEARNING ABOUT ROUTINES: SIX WEEKS TO SIX MONTHS

1 T G R Bower, *A Primer of Infant Development* (Freeman, 1977)
2 The World Health Organization and UNICEF recommend that babies have nothing but breastmilk for the first six months after birth. The Department of Health in England agrees that breastmilk is all a baby needs for the first six months, and recommends that solids not be started before 17 weeks (four months) at the earliest.
3 A Fernald, 'Four-month-old infants prefer to listen to motherese', *Infant Behaviour and Development* 8 (1985): 181–95
4 B E Davis *et al.*, 'Effects of sleep position on infant motor development', *Pediatrics* 102 (1998): 1135–40

4. GETTING SOCIABLE: SIX MONTHS TO TWO YEARS

1 Mary Sheridan, *From Birth to Five Years: Children's Developmental Progress* (Routledge, 1997)
2 Quoted in Deborah Jackson, *Three in a Bed* (Bloomsbury, 1999)
3 S M Bell and M D S Ainsworth, 'Infant Crying and Maternal Responsiveness', *Child Development* 43 (1972): 1171–90
4 E M Ornitz, 'Normal and pathological maturation of vestibular function in the human child', in Romand, *Development of Auditory and Vestibular Systems* (vol 1; Elsevier, 1992): 479–536

5 D L Clark *et al.*, 'Vestibular stimulation influence on motor development in infants', *Science* 196 (1977): 1228–9

5. THE NEED FOR BOUNDARIES

1 For some more resources about boundaries, discipline, etc. I suggest:
Steve Biddulph, *The Secret of Happy Children* (Thorsons, 1999)
Thomas Phelan, *1-2-3 Magic: Training Your Children to Do What You Want* (Child Management Inc, Illinois, 1996)
2 For more on tantrums, try *Toddler Tantrums*, by Penney Hames (Thorsons, 2002)
3 S M Bell and M D S Ainsworth, 'Infant Crying and Maternal Responsiveness', *Child Development* 43 (1972): 1171–90
4 D C van den Boom, 'Behavioral Management of Early Infant Crying in Irritable Babies', in R G Barr, I St James-Roberts and M R Keefe, *New Evidence on Unexplained Early Infant Crying: Its Origins, Nature and Management* (Johnson & Johnson, 2003)
5 Dorothy Einon, *Child Behaviour* (Penguin, 1997)
6 *Ibid.*

Putting the Three-step Plan to Work
Step One: Feeding

6. FEEDING YOUR NEWBORN

1 R Drewett *et al.*, 'From feeds to meals: the development of hunger and food intake in infants and young children', in C Niven and Walker (eds), *Current Issues in Infancy and Parenthood* (Butterworth & Heineman, 1998)
2 P Wright, 'Mothers' assessment of hunger in relation to meal size in breastfeeding infants', *Journal of Reproductive and Infant Psychology* 5 (1987): 173–81

7. HOW MUCH AND HOW OFTEN?

1 Dr Peter Hartmann in Australia is doing this work. See
  http://www.fix.net/~rprewett/evidence.html
  S Daly and P Hartmann, 'Infant Demand and Milk Supply',
  Journal of Human Lactation 11(2) (1995): 21–37
2 *Ibid.*
3 Lisa Marasco and Jan Barger
  http://www.fix.net/~rprewett/evidence.html

8. NIGHT-FEEDING

1 M J Renfrew, S Lang, L Martin, M Woolridge, 'Interventions
  for influencing sleep patterns in exclusively breastfed infants',
  Cochrane Review, Cochrane Library 4 (Oxford, 2001)
2 Wright *et al.*, 'The development of differences in the feeding
  behaviour of bottle and breast fed human infants from birth to
  two months', *Behaviour Process* 5 (1980): 1–20
3 N Butte, 'The evidence for breastfeeding', *Ped Clinc N Amer*
  48.1 (2001): 189–98
4 Two very famous developmental psychologists, L S Vygotsky
  and J Piaget, both identify this as important
5 E Hooker, H L Ball, P J Kelly, 'Sleeping like a baby: attitudes
  and experiences of bedsharing in northeast England', *Med
  Anthropol* 18.3 (2001): 203–22
6 Magda Sachs, 'Sleep Research and Breastfeeding', *BfN
  newsletter* 15 (July 2001)
7 *Ibid.*
8 From notes taken at talk given by Helen Ball at FSID AGM
  Mar 2003, New Scotland Yard

9. YOUR BABY'S NEED TO SUCKLE

1 Brian Palmer, 'Breastfeeding – reducing the risk for obstructive
  sleep apnoea', *Breastfeeding abstracts* 18.3 (1999): 19–20
2 Ros Escott, 'Into the mouths of babes', *Nursing Mothers
  Newsletter*, Christmas 1999

3 'Evidence for the ten steps to successful breastfeeding', WHO (1998)

4 M H Labbok and G E Hendershot, 'Does breastfeeding protect against malocclusion? An analysis of the 1981 Child Health Supplement to the National Health Interview Survey', *American J Preventative Medicine* 3.4 (1987): 227–32

5 C G Zardetto, C R Rodrigues and F M Stefani, 'Effects of different pacifiers on the primary dentition and oral myofunctional structures of preschool children', Pediatr.Dent.24.6 (2002): 552–60

6 'Evidence for the ten steps to successful breastfeeding', WHO (1998)

7 Dr T Berry Brazelton, Touchpoints: *Your Child's Emotional and Behavioural Development* (Penguin, 1992)

8 P Fleming, J Young, A Sawczenko and P Blair, 'Night-time non-nutritive sucking in infants aged 1 to 5 months: relationship with infant state, breastfeeding, and bed-sharing versus room-sharing', *Early Human Development* 56.2–3 (1999): 185–204 – found that routine pacifier users rarely sucked their digits.

9 Alina Tugend, 'To Suck or not to Suck', *New Generation,* June 1996: 16–17

10 Carbajal *et al.*, 'Randomised trial of analgesic effects of sucrose, glucose and pacifiers in term infants', *BMJ* 319 (1999): 1393–7

11 Thanks to Hilary English for this tip!

Step Two: Comfort

10. RECREATING THE WOMB

1 Dr Harvey Karp, *The Happiest Baby on the Block* (Penguin/Michael Joseph, 2002)

2 Lise Eliot, *Early Intelligence* (Penguin, 1999)

3 *Ibid.*

4 *Ibid.*

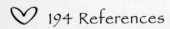

5 *Ibid.*

6 A N Meltzoff and R W Borton, 'Intermodal matching by human neonates', *Nature* 282 (1979): 403–4

7 G F Frederic *et al.*, 'Music Therapy and Pregnancy', *MIDIRS* 12.2 (June 2002): 197–201

8 W S Condon and L W Sander, 'Neonate movement is synchronised with adult speech: Interactional participation and language acquisition', *Science* 183 (1974): 99–101; J Mehler *et al.*, 'A precursor of language acquisition in young infants', *Cognition* 29 (1988): 143–78

9 A J DeCasper and W P Fifer, 'Of Human Bonding – Newborns prefer their mother's voices', *Science* 208 (1980): 1174–76

10 P G Hepper, 'Fetal soap addiction', *Lancet* (June 11, 1988): 1347–8

11 J D Gatts *et al.*, 'Reducing crying and irritability in neonates using a continuously controlled early environment', *J Perinatology* 15.3 (May/June 1995): 215–21

11. USING SOUND AND MOVEMENT

1 G F Frederic *et al.*, 'Music Therapy and Pregnancy', *MIDIRS* 12.2 (June 2002): 197–201

2 Chambers Dictionary

3 Dr Harvey Karp, *The Happiest Baby on the Block* (Penguin/Michael Joseph, 2002)

4 P M Callis, 'The testing and comparison of the intrauterine sound against other methods of calming babies', *Midwives Chronicle* (1984): 336–8

5 A F Korner and E B Thoman, 'Visual alertness in neonates as evoked by maternal care', *J Experimental and Child Psychology* 10 (1970): 67–78

6 V Huhtal *et al.*, 'Infant massage compared with crib vibrator in the treatment of colicky infants', *Pediatrics* 105.6 (June 2000)

7 N Cunningham *et al.*, 'Infant carrying, breastfeeding and mother-infant relations', *Lancet* (February 14, 1987): 379.

Also U A Hunziker and R G Barr, 'Increased carrying reduces infant crying: a randomised controlled trial', *Pediatrics* 77 (1986): 641–8

12. THE POWER OF TOUCH

1 *National Geographic*, November 2002

2 *Ibid.*

3 Paul Martin, *Counting Sheep* (HarperCollins, 2002)

4 Lawrence Stone, *The Family, Sex and Marriage in England 1500–1800* (Penguin, 1977)

5 W and M G Dennis, 'The effects of cradling practices upon the onset of walking in Hopi children', *J Genetic Psychology* 56 (1940): 77–86 – quoted in Lise Eliot, *Early Intelligence* (Penguin, 1999)

6 M C Diamond, 'Evidence for tactile stimulation improving CNS function', in K E Barnard and T B Brazelton (eds), *Touch: The Foundation of Experience* (Madison CT International Universities, 1990): pp 73–96 – quoted in Lise Eliot, *Early Intelligence* (Penguin, 1999)

7 Christensson *et al.*, 'Temperature, metabolic adaptation and crying in healthy fullterm newborns cared for skin-to-skin or in a cot', *Acta paediatrica* 81 (1992): 488–93. Cited in 'Evidence for the ten steps to successful breastfeeding', WHO (1998)

8 Lots of research on this. The Cochrane review supports these findings, though says some studies were methodologically flawed and we cannot extrapolate that massage is a cost-effective treatment. 'Massage for promoting growth and development of preterm and/or low birth-weight infants', *Cochrane Review* (October 1999)

9 Lise Eliot, *Early Intelligence* (Penguin, 1999)

10 V Huhtal *et al.*, 'Infant massage compared with crib vibrator in the treatment of colicky infants', *Pediatrics* 105.6 (June 2000)

13. COMFORTING THE BABY WHO HAS COLIC

1 Tony Long, 'Excessive Infant Crying: how health visitors can help parents', *Community Practitioner* 74.12 (2001): 458–60

2 The original paper was M A Wessel *et al.*, 'Paroxysmal fussing in infancy, sometimes called colic', *Pediatrics* 14 (1954): 421–33. However 'Wessels' rule of threes' is a widely used phrase in the literature

3 R G Barr, 'Colic is something infants do, rather than a condition they have: a developmental approach to crying phenomena, patterns, pacification and (patho)genesis', in R G Barr, I St James-Roberts and M R Keefe, *New Evidence of Unexplained Early Infant Crying: Its Origins, Nature and Management* (Johnson & Johnson, 2003)

4 I St James-Roberts *et al.*, 'Bases for maternal perceptions of infant crying and colic behaviour', *Archives of Disease in Childhood* 75.5 (November 1996): 375–84

5 Sheila Kitzinger, *Crying Baby* (Penguin, 1990). However, some studies have found some medical anomalies in some cases:
   L Lehtonen *et al.*, 'Gallbladder hypocontractility in infantile colic', *Acta Paediatrica* 83.11 (November 1994): 1174–7 found differences in the gallbladder of some babies with colic compared to a control group, and
   L Lothe *et al.*, 'Motilin and infantile colic', *Acta Paediatrica Scandinavica* 79.4 (April 1990): 410–16 – raised levels of motilin from first day of life in infants who develop colic may indicate that the gastrointestinal tract is affected in infants with colic; T Linberg, 'Infantile colic and small intestinal function: a nutritional problem?', *Acta Paediatrica* 88, supplement 430 (August 1999): 58–60; W R Treem, 'Infant colic. A pediatric gastroenterologist's perspective', *Pediatrics Clinics of North America* 41.5 (October 1994): 1121–38

6 M A Hofer, (2003) 'Infant Crying: An evolutionary perspective', in R G Barr *et al.*, *New Evidence of Unexplained Early Infant*

Crying: Its Origins, Nature and Management (Johnson &
Johnson, 2003)

7 From notes on discussion about crying as a developmental
phenomenon in R G Barr *et al.*, *New Evidence of Unexplained
Early Infant Crying: Its Origins, Nature and Management*
(Johnson & Johnson, 2003)

14. FEEDING THE BABY WITH COLIC

1 A Lucas and I St James-Roberts, 'Crying, fussing and colic
behaviour in breast- and bottle-fed infants', *Early Human
Development* 53 (1998): 9–18

2 Tessa Martyn, 'Soya in artificial baby milks', *Practising Midwife*
2.6 (June 1999):16–19

3 B Scach and M Haight, 'Colic and Food Allergy in the Breastfed
infant: Is it possible for an exclusively breastfed infant to suffer
from food allergy?', *J Hum Lact* 18.1 (2002): 50–3

4 J Pincombe and V Thrupp, 'A comparison of crying patterns of
4-week old babies and the effect of zinc supplement in
mothers', *Australian College of Midwives Incorporated Journal*
13.4 (December 2000): 15–21

5 K D Lust *et al.*, 'Maternal intake of cruciferous vegetables and
other foods and colic symptoms in exclusively breastfed infants',
J American Dietetic Association 96.1 (January 1996): 46–8

6 T Lindberg, 'Infantile colic and small intestinal function: a
nutritional problem?', *Acta Paediatrica* 88 supplement 430
(August 1999): 58–60; I Jakobsson *et al.*, 'Effectiveness of
casein hydrolysate feedings in infants with colic', *Acta
Paediatrica* 89.1 (January 2000): 18–21

7 L Lothe and T Lindberg, 'Cow's milk whey protein elicits
symptoms of infantile colic in colicky formula-fed infants: a
double-blind crossover study', *Pediatrics* 83.2 (February 1989):
262–6

8 C and L Lawlor-Smith, 'Lactose Intolerance', *Breastfeeding
Review* 6.1 (1998): 29–30

9 Joy Anderson, 'Lactose Intolerance and the breastfed baby',
   Nursing Mothers Newsletter (Summer 1999): 4–6. Also M
   Woolridge, 'Colic, "Overfeeding" and symptoms of Lactose
   Malabsorption in the Breastfed infant: a possible artifact of
   feed management?', *Lancet* (August 13, 1988): 382–4
10 Evans *et al.* (1995), cited in Renfrew *et al.*, *Enabling Women to
   breastfeed* (HMSO, 2000)
11 M Woolridge *et al.*, 'Do changes in pattern of breast usage alter
   the baby's nutrient intake?', *Lancet* 336 (August 18, 1990):
   395–7

15. IS YOUR COLICKY BABY OVERSENSITIVE?

1 Research findings quoted and summarized in Sheila Kitzinger,
   Crying Baby (Penguin, 1990); also A R Miller, R G Barr and
   W O Eaton, 'Crying and motor behaviour of six-week-old
   infants and postpartum maternal mood', *Pediatrics* 92.4
   (October 1993): 551–8 – Clinically significant levels of crying
   (or colic) are differentially associated with different patterns of
   clinically significant maternal distress – possible indicator of
   stressed mother-infant relationship.
2 R G Barr *et al.*, 'Crying patterns in pre-term infants',
   Developmental medicine and child neurology 38.4 (April 1996):
   345–55
3 *Ibid.*
4 T J Clifford *et al.*, '(2002) Infant colic: empirical evidence of
   the absence of an association with source of early infant
   nutrition', *Arch. Pediatr. Adolesc. Med.* 156(11): 1123–8
5 P Rautava *et al.*, 'Psychosocial predisposing factors for infantile
   colic', *BMJ* 307.6904 (4 September 1993): 600–4
6 C Sondergaard *et al.*, 'Fetal growth and infantile colic', *Archives
   of disease in childhood (fetal and neonatal edition)*, 83.1 (July
   2000): 44–7

7 J W Crawford, 'Mother-infant interaction in premature and full-term infants', *Child Development* 53 (1982): 957–62, quoted in Sheila Kitzinger, *Crying Baby* (Penguin, 1990)

8 M R Keef *et al.*, 'Newborn predictors of infant irritability', *J Obstetric, Gynecologic and Neonatal Nursing* 27.5 (September/October 1998): 513–20

9 I St James-Roberts and P Menon-Johansson, 'Predicting infant crying from fetal movement data: an exploratory study', *Early Human Development* 54.1 (February 1999): 55–62

10 Nancy Morgan, 'Strategies for Colic', *Birth Gazette* 12.4 (Fall 1996)

11 Dr T Berry Brazelton, *Touchpoints: Your Child's Emotional and Behavioural Development* (Penguin, 1992)

12 Nathan Fox and Cindy Polak, 'The possible contribution of temperament to understanding the origins and consequences of persistent and excessive crying', in R G Barr *et al.*, *New Evidence of Unexplained Early Infant Crying: Its Origins, Nature and Management* (Johnson & Johnson, 2003)

13 Dr T Berry Brazelton, *Touchpoints: Your Child's Emotional and Behavioural Development* (Penguin, 1992)

14 R G Barr *et al.*, 'Effects of intra-oral sucrose on crying, mouthing and hand-mouth contact in newborn and six-week-old infants', *Developmental Medicine and Child Neurology* 36.7 (July 1994): 608–18

15 R G Barr, S N Young *et al.*, 'Differential calming responses to sucrose taste in crying infants with and without colic', *Pediatrics* 103.5 (May 1999)

16 T Markestad, 'Use of sucrose as a treatment for infant colic', *Archives of Disease in Childhood* 76.4 (April 1997): 356–8

17 Six-week grizzle – randomized controlled trial – carrying babies for an extra two hours a day from three weeks onwards resulted them in crying less than babies who were not carried around like this. Hunziker and Barr, 'Increased carrying reduces infant crying', *Pediatrics* 77 (1986): 641–8

♡ 200 References

18 R G Barr et al., 'Carrying as colic "therapy": a randomised controlled trial', Pediatrics 87.5 (May 1991): 623–30

19 I St James-Roberts et al., 'Supplementary carrying compared with advice to increase responsive parenting as interventions to prevent infant crying', Pediatrics 95.3 (March 1995): 381–8

16. TREATMENTS FOR COLIC

1 M Garrison et al., 'A systematic review of treatments for infantile colic', Pediatrics 106.1 (July 2000):184–90; Teresa Kilgour and Sally Wade, 'Infantile Colic', Clin Evid (2002): 321–30

2 Pinyerd (1992), quoted in Nancy Morgan, 'Strategies for Colic', Birth Gazette 12.4 (Fall 1996)

3 T J Metcalf et al., 'Simethicone in the treatment of infant colic: a randomised placebo-controlled multicenter trial', Pediatrics 94.1 (July 1994): 29–34

4 M Garrison et al., 'A systematic review of treatments for infantile colic', Pediatrics 106.1 (July 2000):184–90

5 C J Hayden, 'Towards an Understanding of Osteopathy in the treatment of infantile colic', J Manual and Manipulative Therapy (2002): 162

6 J Wiberg et al., 'The short-term effect of spinal manipulation in the treatment of infantile colic: a randomised controlled clinical trial with a blinded observer', J Manipulative and Physiological Therapeutics 22.8 (October 1999): 517–22. Abstracted and commented on in MIDIRS December 2000: 514–15

7 E Olafsdottir et al., 'Randomised controlled trial of infantile colic treated with chiropractic spinal manipulation', Archives of Disease in Childhood 84.2 (February 2001): 138–41, abstracted and commented on in MIDIRS 2001 (ref 20010313-29) by Lou Bashall chiropractor and Christine Andrew chiropractor/midwife

8 Nancy Morgan, 'Strategies for Colic', Birth Gazette 12.4 (Fall 1996)

9 M Garrison *et al.*, 'A systematic review of treatments for infantile colic', *Pediatrics* 106.1 (July 2000):184-90

Step Three: Sleeping

17. HOW SLEEP WORKS FOR YOU

1 Owen Flanagan, *Dreaming Souls Sleep, Dreams and the Evolution of the Conscious Mind* (Oxford University Press, 2000)
2 Paul Martin, *Counting Sheep* (HarperCollins, 2001)
3 William Sears, *Nighttime Parenting* (Penguin, 1999)
4 Dilys Daws, *Through the Night* (Free Association Books, 1993)

18. HOW SLEEP WORKS FOR YOUR BABY

1 William Sears, *Nighttime Parenting* (Penguin, 1999)
2 Ruth Martin, in *Before the Baby and After* (1958), quotes that mothers could expect their babies to sleep for 21 to 24 hours a day for the first two months – in Christina Hardyment, *ibid.*
3 James J McKenna, 'Sudden Infant Death Syndrome in Cross-Cultural Perspective: Is Infant-Parent cosleeping protective?', *Ann. Rev. Anthropol.* 25 (1996): 201–16
4 B R H van den Bergh, 'Maternal emotions during pregnancy and fetal neonatal behaviour,' in J G Nijhuis (ed), *Fetal Behaviour: Developmental and Perinatal Aspects* (NYU/Oxford University Press, 1992): 157–78
5 A M Walker, S Menahem, 'Normal early infant behaviour patterns', *J Paediatrics and Child Health* 30.3 (June 1994): 260–2
6 K A Freudigman, E B Thman, 'Infants' earliest sleep/wake organisation differs as a function of delivery mode', *Dev Psychobiol* 32.4 (May 1998): 292–303
7 David Messer and Carol Parker, 'Infants' sleep: patterns and problems', in Catherine Niven and Anne Walker (eds), *Current Issues in Infancy and Parenthood* (Butterworth-Heineman, 1998)
8 Paul Martin, *Counting Sheep* (HarperCollins, 2001)

♡ 202 References

19. CAN YOU TRAIN YOUR BABY TO SLEEP THROUGH THE NIGHT?

1 David Messer and Carol Parker, 'Infants' sleep: patterns and problems', in Catherine Niven and Anne Walker (eds), *Current Issues in Infancy and Parenthood* (Butterworth-Heineman, 1998)
2 *Ibid.*
3 P Ramchandani *et al.*, 'A systematic review of treatments for settling problems and night-waking in young children', *BMJ* 320 (22 January 2000): 209–13
4 David Messer and Carol Parker, 'Infants' sleep: patterns and problems', in Catherine Niven and Anne Walker (eds), *Current Issues in Infancy and Parenthood* (Butterworth-Heineman, 1998)

20. HELPING YOUR BABY FALL ASLEEP

1 M Nikolopoulou, I St James-Roberts, 'Preventing sleeping problems in infants who are at risk of developing them', *Arch Dis Child* 88.2 (2003): 108–11; M J Renfrew *et al.*, 'Interventions for influencing sleep patterns in exclusively breastfed infants', *Cochrane Review*, Cochrane Library Issue 4 (2001), Oxford; T Pinella, L Birch, 'Help me make it through the night: behavioural entrainment of breastfed infants' sleep patterns', *Pediatrics* 91.2 (February 1993): 436–44
2 Paul Martin, *Counting Sheep* (HarperCollins, 2001)

21. HELPING YOUR BABY STAY ASLEEP

1 I St James-Roberts *et al.*, 'Use of a behavioural programme in the first three months to prevent infant crying and sleeping problems', *J Paediatr. Child Health* 37 (2001): 289–97
2 B Hollyer and L Smith, *Sleep: The Secret of Problem-free Nights* (WardLock, 1996)
3 I St James-Roberts *et al.*, 'Use of a behavioural programme in the first three months to prevent infant crying and sleeping problems', *J Paediatr. Child Health* 37 (2001): 289–97
4 *Ibid.*

22. ALL CHANGE: SLEEP AND THE OLDER BABY

1 Jenkins *et al.*, 'Continuities of common behaviour problems in preschool children', *J Child Psychology and Psychiatry* 25 (1984): 75–89

23. WHO SLEEPS WHERE?

1 Paul Martin, *Counting Sheep* (HarperCollins, 2001)

2 James McKenna, 'Breastfeeding and bedsharing', *Mothering* (September/October 2002)

3 F P Pankhurst and J A Horne, 'Influence of bed partners on movement during sleep', *Sleep* 17 (1994): 308

4 James McKenna and Sarah Mosko, 'Co-sleeping mothers and infants influence sleep physiology: overview and implications', *Proceedings of the Third Congress of the European Society for the Study and Prevention of Infant Deaths* (Oxford: John Radcliffe, August 1993); James McKenna *et al.*, 'Experimental studies of infant-parent co-sleeping: mutual physiological and behavioural influences and their relevance to SIDS (sudden infant death syndrome)', *Early Human Development* 38 (1994) 187–201

5 Cory A Mermer response to Blair *et al.*, 'Babies sleeping with parents: case-control study of factors influencing the risk of the sudden infant death syndrome', *BMJ* 319 (4 December 1999): 1457–62. Commentary is by Ed Mitchell, Associate Professor in Paediatrics – http://bmj.com/cgi/content/full/319/7223/1457

6 Dilys Daws, *Through the Night* (Free Association Books, 1989)

7 M F Elias *et al.*, 'Sleep/wake patterns of breastfed infants in the first two years of life', *Pediatrics* 77.3 (March 1986): 322–9; Magda Sachs, 'Sleep Research and Breastfeeding', *BfN newsletter* 15 (July 2001)

8 E Hooker, H L Ball, P J Kelly, 'Sleeping like a baby: attitudes and experiences of bedsharing in northeast England', *Med Anthropol* 18.3 (2001): 203–22

9 http://www.dur.ac.uk/~dcm0www/DF/sleeplab.htm

10 Deborah Jackson, *Three in a Bed* (Bloomsbury, 1999)

11 P Fleming *et al.*, 'Sudden unexpected deaths in infancy', The CESDI/SUDI series (The Stationery Office, February 2000)

12 Hugh Jolly, *Book of Child Care* (Unwin, 1985)

13 Wolf, Lozoff, and Davis, 'Cosleeping in urban families with young children in the United States', *Pediatrics* 72 (1984): 171–82

24. SLEEPING SAFELY

1 http://www.sids.org.uk/fsid/cot.htm

2 *Ibid.*

3 *Ibid.*

4 James McKenna *et al.*, 'Experimental studies of infant-parent co-sleeping: mutual physiological and behavioural influences and their relevance to SIDS (sudden infant death syndrome)', *Early Human Development* 38 (1994): 187–201

5 James J McKenna, 'Sudden Infant Death Syndrome in Cross-Cultural Perspective: Is Infant-Parent co-sleeping protective?', *Ann.Rev. Anthropol.* 25 (1996): 201–16

6 *Ibid.*

7 Commentary on Blair *et al.*, 'Babies sleeping with parents: case-control study of factors influencing the risk of the sudden infant death syndrome', *BMJ* 319 (4 December 1999): 1457–62. Commentary is by Ed Mitchell, Associate Professor in Paediatrics – http://bmj.com/cgi/content/full/319/7223/1457

8 B Alm *et al.*, 'Breastfeeding and the sudden infant death syndrome in Scandinavia, 1992–5', *Archives of Disease in Childhood* 86 (2002): 400–2

9 H Zotter, R Kerbl, R Kurz, W Muller, 'Pacifier use and sudden infant death syndrome: should health professionals recommend pacifier use based on present knowledge?', *Wien.Klin.Wochenschr.* 114.17–18 (2002): 791–4

10 Commentary on Blair *et al.*, 'Babies sleeping with parents: case-control study of factors influencing the risk of the sudden infant death syndrome', *BMJ* 319 (4 December 1999):

1457–62. Commentary is by Ed Mitchell, Associate Professor in Paediatrics – http://bmj.com/cgi/content/full/319/7223/1457

11 *Ibid.*

12 Peter Fleming, public talk reported in *La Leche League Great Britain News*

13 *BabyZone,* Foundation for the Study of Infant Deaths, 2003

14 D Tappin *et al.,* 'Used infant mattresses and sudden infant death syndrome in Scotland: case-control study', *BMJ* 325.7371 (2002): 1007–12

15 'Clean mattresses for babies' *FSID news* (Spring 2003)

16 James J McKenna, 'Sudden Infant Death Syndrome in Cross-Cultural Perspective: Is Infant-Parent co-sleeping protective?', *Ann.Rev. Anthropol.* 25 (1996): 201–16

17 R Neunteufl, F Eichler, M Urschitz, M Tiefenthaler, 'Does professional counseling improve infant home monitoring? Evaluation of an intensive instruction program for families using home monitoring on their babies', *Wien.Klin.Wochenschr.* 114.17-18 (2002): 801–6

18 Commentary on Blair *et al.,* 'Babies sleeping with parents: case-control study of factors influencing the risk of the sudden infant death syndrome', *BMJ* 319 (4 December 1999): 1457–62. Commentary is by Ed Mitchell, Associate Professor in Paediatrics – http://bmj.com/cgi/content/full/319/7223/1457

19 Deborah Jackson, *Three in a Bed* (Bloomsbury, 1998)

20 James McKenna *et al.,* 'Experimental studies of infant-parent co-sleeping: mutual physiological and behavioural influences and their relevance to SIDS (sudden infant death syndrome)', *Early Human Development* 38 (1994): 187–201

21 *Ibid.*

22 *Ibid.*

23 James McKenna and Sarah Mosko, 'Co-sleeping mothers and infants influence sleep physiology: overview and implications', *Proceedings of the Third Congress of the European Society for the Study and Prevention of Infant Deaths* (Oxford: John Radcliffe, August 1993)

24 Deborah Jackson, *Three in a Bed* (Bloomsbury, 1999)
25 James J McKenna, 'Sudden Infant Death Syndrome in Cross-Cultural Perspective: Is Infant-Parent co-sleeping protective?', *Ann.Rev. Anthropol.* 25 (1996): 201–16
26 Quote from Notre Dame's Website, Notre Dame University, Indiana, USA: http:www.nd.edu/
27 James McKenna and Sarah Mosko, 'Co-sleeping mothers and infants influence sleep physiology: overview and implications', *Proceedings of the Third Congress of the European Society for the Study and Prevention of Infant Deaths* (Oxford: John Radcliffe, August 1993)
28 James McKenna *et al.*, 'Experimental studies of infant-parent co-sleeping: mutual physiological and behavioural influences and their relevance to SIDS (sudden infant death syndrome)', *Early Human Development* 38 (1994): 187–201

25. PUTTING IT ALL TOGETHER: WHAT'S GOING TO WORK FOR YOU?

1 Paul Martin, *Counting Sheep* (HarperCollins, 2002)
2 Dilys Daws, *Through the Night* (Free Association Books, 1989)
3 Notes at a talk given by Helen Ball at FSIDs AGM, March 2003, at New Scotland Yard

Useful Organizations
and Further Reading

Serene/CRY-sis
Support for families with excessively crying, sleepless and demanding children.
BM CRY-sis
London WC1N 3XX
CRY-sis helpline 0207 404 5011
Operates from 8am to 11pm, seven days a week

ParentlinePlus
Support and information for all families (incorporating Parent Network courses on parenting skills).
ParentlinePlus
520 Highgate Studios
53-79 Highgate Road
Kentish Town
London NW5 1TL
Helpline 0207 284 5000
www.parentlineplus.org.uk

Meet-A-Mum Association (MAMA)
MAMA organizes local groups offering friendship and support to
mothers who feel isolated or have postnatal depression.
Helpline 0208 768 0123
Operates from 7pm to 10pm weekday evenings
10am to 1pm on Mondays and Wednesdays

The Foundation for the Study of Infant Deaths (FSID)
Information about avoiding cot death.
FSID
Artillery House
11-19 Artillery Row
London SW1P 1RT
Tel: 0207 222 8001
Fax: 0207 222 8002
www.sids.org.uk/fsid/

Child Psychotherapy Trust
The CPT have a series of leaflets on emotional development and
baby behaviour, and relationships to parents, such as 'Your New
Baby' and 'Crying and Sleeping'. These cost £1 each and are
available from the CPT at:
Child Psychotherapy Trust
Star House
104-108 Grafton Road
London NW5 4BD
Tel: 0207 284 1355
E-mail: cpt@globalnet.co.uk
Please enclose an A4 SAE to cover postage.

The Brazelton Neonatal Behavioural Assessment Scale
Dr Joanna Hawthorne
The Brazelton Centre in Great Britain
c/o Box 226
Addenbrooke's NHS Trust
Hills Road
Cambridge
CB2 2QQ
Tel: 01223 245791
www.brazelton.co.uk

The Brazelton Neonatal Behavioural Assessment Scale is a clinical exercise that can be carried out with a new baby at any time from birth to two months of age. A trained assessor will examine all the baby's capabilities and discuss them with his or her parents. It can be particularly useful where there is any anxiety on the part of the parents or worry about the baby's progress.

The NBAS was first put together by US paediatrician Dr T Berry Brazelton. You can find out more information about the Brazelton NBAS at the website above.

Complementary Practitioners

ACUPUNCTURE
For a list of registered acupuncturists who have trained to work with children, contact:
June Tranmer MBAcC
Practitioner of Paediatric Acupuncture
The Healing Clinic
33 Fulford Cross
York YO10 4PB
Tel: 01904 679868

CRANIAL OSTEOPATHY
Osteopathic Centre for Children
109 Harley Street
London W1G 6AN
Tel: 0207 486 6160

HOMOEOPATHY
For a full list of doctors trained in homoeopathy, an information
pack and NHS availability, send an SAE to:
British Homoeopathic Association
15 Clerkenwell Close
London EC1R 5AA
Tel: 0207 566 7800

BABY MASSAGE
For details of baby massage classes and qualified baby masseurs
near you, contact:
International Association of Infant Massage (UK Office)
56 Sparsholt Road,
Barking
Essex IG11 7YQ
Tel: 07816 289788
From 10.30am to 2.30pm
www.iaim.org.uk

The Guild of Infant and Child Massage
Tel: 07796 916179
www.gicm.org.uk

International Association of Infant Massage
Tel: 07816 289788

See also www.touchneeds.com
Tel: 01889 560260

Further Reading

Steve Biddulph, *Secrets of Happy Children* (Thorsons, 1998)
Lise Eliot, *Early Intelligence* (Penguin, 1999)
Deborah Jackson, *Three in a Bed* (Bloomsbury, 1998)
Paul Martin, *Counting Sheep* (HarperCollins, 2002)
Asha Phillips, *Saying No* (Faber & Faber, 1999)

Other Books from NCT Publishing:

Caroline Deacon, *Breastfeeding for Beginners*
Penney Hames, *Help Your Baby to Sleep*
Penney Hames, *Toddler Tantrums*
Ravinder Lilly, *First Foods*
Heather Welford, *Successful Potty Training*
The NCT Complete Book of Baby Care

All available from NCT Maternity Sales: 0870 112 1120 or
www.nctms.co.uk

All about the National Childbirth Trust

The National Childbirth Trust wants all parents to have an experience of pregnancy, birth and early parenthood that enriches their lives and gives them confidence in being a parent.

National Childbirth Trust
Alexandra House
Oldham Terrace
London W3 6NH

Run by parents, for parents, the National Childbirth Trust is a self-help charity organization with 400 branches across the UK. There's bound to be a local branch near you, running

- **childbirth classes**
- **breastfeeding counselling**
- **new baby groups**
- **open house get-togethers**
- **support for dads**
- **working parents' groups**
- **nearly-new sales of baby clothes and equipment**

– as well as loads of events where you can meet and make friends with other people going through the same changes.

To find the contact details of your local branch, ring the NCT Enquiry Line: 0870 444 8707

To get support with feeding your baby, ring the NCT Breastfeeding Line: 0870 444 8708

To find answers to pregnancy queries, ring the Enquiry Line or log on to: www.nctpregnancyandbabycare.com

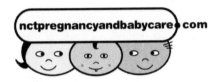

To buy excellent baby goods, maternity bras, toys and gifts, look at:

www.nctms.co.uk or telephone 0870 112 1120.

To join the NCT, just call 0870 990 8040.

You don't have to become a member to enjoy the services and support of the National Childbirth Trust. It's open to everyone. We do encourage people to join the charity because it helps fund our work – supporting all parents.

When you become an NCT member and join your local group, you'll get a regular neighbourhood newsletter (a guide to the area aimed at new parents) and you'll also receive NCT's New Generation – our mailed out members' magazine that takes an in-depth look at all issues of interest to new parents.

If you have a computer that's connected to the internet, you can also join one of our e-groups. There's your 'NCT Coffee Morning' at:

http://groups.yahoo.com/group/nct-coffee/

and there's support for parents of premature babies at:

http://groups.yahoo.com/group/nct-preterm

and support for women recovering from a caesarean at:

http://groups.yahoo.com/group/nct-caesarean

The NCT support network is second to none. It's very reassuring and comforting.

– Kerry

Index

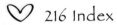

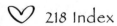

intelligence
  breastfeeding and 55
  carrying and 27
  mothers' responsiveness and 6
  sleep and 118
  touch and 81

Jackson, Deborah 163, 173

kissing 59
Kitzinger, Sheila 100

lactase 94
lactose intolerance 94
lactose overload 95–6
language
  foetuses and 70
  'proto-conversation' 18
learning theory *see* behaviourism
Lester, Barry 4, 6
'let-down reflex' 86
listening, in the womb 71
lullabies 75
lying-in 10–11

malocclusion 60, 61, 62
margarines, milk-free 184
massage 81–2
mattresses, second-hand 170–1
McKenna, James 123, 172–3,
  174
milk substitutes 187
monitors 171–2
Moro (startle) reflex 69, 80

'motherese' 20
movement
  and comfort 20, 75–7
  in the womb 69
music 70, 74–5, 77

naps *see* daytime naps
NCT National Breastfeeding Line
  13
newborns 10–16
  comfort 14
  feeding 12–13, 41–52
  sleep 14–15, 123–4
'night treats' 155
night-feeding 53–8, 146
night terrors 154
nightmares 154
non-rapid-eye-movement
  (NREM) sleep
  adults 116–17
  babies 125
  newborns 123, 124

'obligatory looking' 18
Odent, Michael 26
over-heating 170
overlaying 163
overtiredness
  and colic 99–100
  toddlers 152

pain
  colic and 85–6
  crying and 7–8

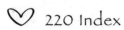

Make
www.thorsonselement.com
your online sanctuary

Get online information, inspiration and
guidance to help you on the path to physical
and spiritual well-being. Drawing on the integrity
and vision of our authors and titles, and with
health advice, articles, astrology, tarot, a
meditation zone, author interviews and events
listings, www.thorsonselement.com is a great
alternative to help create space and peace
in our lives.

So if you've always wondered about practising
yoga, following an allergy-free diet, using the
tarot or getting a life coach, we can point you
in the right direction.

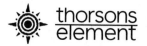
thorsons
element